Mapping the Edges and the In-between
A critical analysis of borderline personality disorder

International Perspectives in Philosophy and Psychiatry

Series editors: KWM (Bill) Fulford, Katherine Morris, John Z Sadler, and Giovanni Stanghellini

Volumes in the series:

Mapping the Edges and the In-between

A critical analysis of borderline personality disorder

Edited by

Nancy Nyquist Potter

Professor of Philosophy,
University of Louisville;
President, Association for the
Advancement of Philosophy and
Psychiatry,
University of Louisville

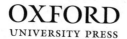

OXFORD
UNIVERSITY PRESS

OXFORD
UNIVERSITY PRESS

Great Clarendon Street, Oxford OX2 6DP

Oxford University Press is a department of the University of Oxford.
It furthers the University's objective of excellence in research, scholarship,
and education by publishing worldwide in

Oxford New York

Auckland Cape Town Dar es Salaam Hong Kong Karachi
Kuala Lumpur Madrid Melbourne Mexico City Nairobi
New Delhi Shanghai Taipei Toronto

With offices in

Argentina Austria Brazil Chile Czech Republic France Greece
Guatemala Hungary Italy Japan Poland Portugal Singapore
South Korea Switzerland Thailand Turkey Ukraine Vietnam

Oxford is a registered trade mark of Oxford University Press
in the UK and in certain other countries

Published in the United States
by Oxford University Press Inc., New York

British Library Cataloguing in Publication Data

Data available

Library of Congress Cataloging in Publication Data

Data available

Typeset in Minion
by Cepha Imaging Private Ltd., Bangalore, India
Printed in Great Britain
on acid-free paper by the
MPG Books Group, Bodmin and King's Lynn

ISBN 978–0–19–853021–3 (pbk)

10 9 8 7 6 5 4 3 2 1

Dedicated to
Rif, teacher, mentor, humorist
and
Rob, beloved and friend

Contents

Acknowledgements

The author would like to thank the following for permission to use previously published excerpts of her work:

Potter, N. (1996). Discretionary power, lies, and broken trust: Justification and discomfort. *Theoretical Medicine and Bioethics*, **17**(4): 329–352.

Potter, N. (1996). Loopholes, gaps, and what is held fast: Democratic epistemology and claims to recovered memories. *Philosophy, Psychiatry, and Psychology*, **3**(4): 237–254.

Potter, N. (2000). Giving uptake. *Social Theory and Practice*, **Fall 2000**, **26**(3): 479–508.

Potter, N. (2002). *How can I be Trusted? A Virtue Theory of Trustworthiness.* Maryland, New York, and Oxford: Rowman-Littlefield.

Potter, N. (2002) Can prisoners learn victim empathy? An analysis of a relapse prevention program in the Kentucky State Reformatory for Men. In N. Potter (ed), *Putting Peace into Practice: Evaluating Policy on Local and Global Levels*, 55–75. Amsterdam: Rodopi Press.

Potter, N. (2003). Commodity/Body/Sign: Borderline Personality Disorder and the signification of self-injurious behavior. *Philosophy, Psychiatry, and Psychology*, **10**(1): 1–16.

Potter, N. (2003). Moral tourists and 'world'-travelers: Some epistemological considerations for understanding patients' worlds. *Philosophy, Psychiatry, and Psychology*, **10**(3): 209–223.

Potter, N. (2005). Liberatory psychiatry and an ethics of the in-between. In: M. Shildrick and R. Mykitiuk (eds), *Ethics of the Body: Postconventional Challenges*, 113–133. Cambridge, Mass: MIT Press.

Potter, N. (2006).What is manipulative behavior, anyway? *Journal of Personality Disorders* **20**(2): 139–156.

Potter, N. (2008). The problem with too much anger: A philosophical approach to understanding anger in borderline personality disordered patients. In L. Charland and P. Zachar (eds), *Fact and Value in Emotion*, 53–64. Amsterdam: John Benjamins.

Introduction

I first became interested in borderline personality disorder (BPD) when I worked as a certified Crisis Counselor for 5 years in a large metropolitan city. After having decided to change my degree plan from clinical psychology to philosophy, I wanted to be sure that I stayed grounded in ordinary life problems; philosophy has a reputation for being esoteric, abstract, and largely irrelevant. This was in the mid-1980s, when the BPD diagnosis was fairly new, and I was sometimes warned not to be engaged with a particular crisis client because 'she was a borderline.' I was dismayed and puzzled by the derision and dismissal some of my colleagues were expressing, but I determined to understand what lay beneath it. Thus, I launched my passion about the diagnosis, the people who are diagnosed with it, and those who work with these patients.

This introduction will serve to orient the reader to this diagnosis, my methodology, and the aims of this book. I'll begin by situating BPD within the field of psychiatry.

(i) What is it? Who has it? Axis II and the Cluster B personality disorders

Personality theory is rich and diverse (cf. Pervin and John 1999), but the general idea of personality is that it is the 'characteristic manner in which one thinks, feels, behaves, and relates to others' (Widiger *et al*. 1999, p. 347). It includes the cognitions, affects, and behaviors that are patterned and organized (both conscious and unconscious ones) and that tend to shape the direction of one's choices and life-plans (Cross and Markus 1999, p. 382). A personality disorder, by contrast, is a structural organization of the personality that is exhibited by a dysfunctional pattern of behavior. A personality disorder is stable over time and, because it is a structural defect in internal organization, it is considered to be inflexible. The inner experience of a personality disorder, along with its outward manifestations, causes the person distress or impairment in functioning (cf. DSM-IV-TR 2000; Millon 1996).

BPD is one of several mental illnesses that come under the heading of personality disorders. Personality disorders are considered to be long-standing structural flaws in personality that are inflexible and maladaptive, creating problems in living.[1] The PDs are considered more severe and less likely to recover from than mental disorders – those found in Axis I – and so are categorized differently. According to Theodore Millon, the Axis II model considers the entire matrix of the person, and pathologies that are found in personalities are not considered diseases; diseases belong on Axis I (Millon 1996, p. 190.) The Axis II category includes 10 personality disorders and mental retardation. Within the categorization of PDs, there exist subsets consisting of Cluster A PDs (that display odd or eccentric behavior), the Cluster Bs (that are marked by dramatic or erratic behavior), and the Cluster Cs (those marked by anxious or inhibited behavior). As Millon points out, Axis II together with Axis IV, the psychosocial environment, may produce Axis I mental disorders; hence, the value of a multiaxial framework is that it takes into account the broader context in which we live (Millon 1996, p. 136).

The borderline personality is classified under the Cluster B personality disorders. It is characterized by identity disturbance, feelings of chronic emptiness, impulsive or self-destructive behavior, and unstable intense interpersonal relationships. Other key characteristics include a loss of a sense of self separate from others, contradictory self-images that are experienced as an inner void and an abundance of mismanaged anger. Distrust, all-or-nothing thinking, extreme sensitivity to perceptions of unfair treatment, and an appearance of normality that quickly unravels under stress are additional features.

A significant percentage of the population in the Western world is diagnosed with this personality disorder: 10% of the patients seen in outpatient mental health facilities and 20% of those seen as psychiatric inpatients are diagnosed with BPD (American Psychiatric Association (APA) 2000). These patients experience dysphoria more intensely and for longer periods than other psychiatric patients (Zanarini et al. 1998), living lives that are painful and distressing. Furthermore, BPD is about five times more common among first-degree biological relatives of those diagnosed with BPD than among the general population. When the ethics of treatment are closely examined and the results of that examination incorporated into practice, patients are more likely to stay in treatment. Good treatment – that is, therapeutically and ethically good – should also have a positive effect on families at risk, thus decreasing the likelihood that the next generation will develop symptoms of BPD.

---

[1] See my 'Perplexing issues in personality disorders' for a discussion of co-morbidity within the personality disorders and concerns about the proliferation of them (Potter 2004).

(ii) **The hand-in-hand philosophical and clinical work to be done**

This is a population at risk; patients diagnosed with BPD have a reputation for being extremely difficult to work with. Indeed, clinicians often self-report attitudes of blame, rejection, and a lack of empathy for BPD patients. But this book is important not only for its emphasis on moral psychology for mental health professionals but also intellectually. I'll start with the conceptual issues.

The criteria for diagnosis of BPD raise difficult philosophical questions. For example, impulsive behavior is a characteristic not only of many BPD patients, but also of bipolar patients, people with addictions, and adolescents. Being impulsive is generally regarded as irrational – unwise at best, self-destructive at its worst. But what exactly is impulsivity? Can we be impulsive and still reason well? How do concepts such as the will and deliberation address questions about impulsivity? How is impulsivity different from spontaneity? Why is being impulsive usually regarded as a character defect whereas being spontaneous is not? Are clinicians clear about where the line is drawn between impulsivity and spontaneity? What difference might it make to clinical practice if the philosophical underpinnings of impulsivity, deliberation, and willing were better understood?

Not only are concepts such impulsivity under-examined; when it comes to personality disorders, epistemic inquiry tends to be suspended on crucial questions such as what counts as healthy self-concepts, healthy decision-making, and healthy interpersonal relationships. A view of mental health that includes a unified self with stable relationships and moods, a coherent sense of past and future, and an ability to be a responsible and deliberate decision-maker leads to the assessment of those who dispositionally fail to exhibit or experience such a self as unhealthy. What is the metaphysical and epistemological status of this view of the self? Is it reliable as a standard against which to measure such things as identity disturbance or extreme aggression and anger? How significant a role do cultural values and ideologies play in shaping assessments of people whose behavior departs from mental health norms? Does gendered socialization affect how men and women differ in their experience of self and how they negotiate anger?

Assumptions about healthy selves and personalities, combined with clinician attitudes that BPD patients are people to be warned about and suspicious of, require careful and minute analysis. Cultural factors and social norms play a significant role in all of our behaviors and how those behaviors are interpreted, and the diagnosis and treatment of patients with symptoms of BPD are no exception (cf. Paris 1996.) In fact, the construct of BPD arguably obscures the clinical picture of patients given this diagnosis instead of clarifying it (Crowe 2004). It is possible that some of our deeply held ideas about the self, identity, anger, and so on lead us astray when we interact with others in distress, attempt to interpret their behavior, and respond to their communications. It is also possible that some of the concepts that we rely upon (such as manipulativity) are too vague to serve as a basis of ethically responsive and therapeutically constructive clinical work. A central task of this book, then, is to press questions of to what extent the symptoms of the classificatory disorder BPD represent pathology or, instead, cultural disapproval or social disvalue – what is often called the 'mad or bad' problem. This problem points to a difficulty in determining whether a given diagnosis is genuinely psychiatric in character or is indicative of embedded moral values that do not belong to psychiatric judgment. This theme is threaded throughout the book but is most directly treated in Chapter 9, when I complete Part II on virtues relevant to treatment with BPD patients. A philosophical and clinically informed analysis allows me to develop a treatment ethics that corrects some of the assumptions that underlie current approaches to treatment of patients diagnosed with BPD. Finally, this project can provide readers with conceptual tools to use for diagnosis and nosology.

Characteristics that BPD patients bring to the clinical setting make treatment particularly rocky and tumultuous. Clinicians typically find therapeutic work with BPD patients to be difficult and frustrating, and they tend to discuss BPD patients in terms of warnings and cautions. In fact, although the term 'borderline' has historically marked a boundary between psychotic and neurotic personality types, it has increasingly come into usage as a noun that carries a pejorative meaning. This can be seen in language used to describe treatment of such patients. They are considered difficult to treat because of 'the intensity of their engagement with caregivers, the sometimes overwhelming nature of their demands for care, and the strong emotions and conflicts that they provoke in others' (Herman *et al.* 1989). Put less delicately, one researcher claims to distinguish BPD patients from depressed or schizophrenic ones by 'their angry, demanding, and entitled presentation,' and another warns that 'any interviewer, whether with a clinical or research purpose, will be exposed to devaluation, manipulation, angry outbursts, clinging or appeal' (Mitton and Huxley 1988). Most bluntly, 'borderliners are the patients you think of as PIAs – pains in the ass,' as a past chairman of the psychiatry department at New York University put it (*Medical World News* 1983).

We might ask, 'What is it about BPD patients that makes treatment so rocky?' Or to put it differently, 'What is it about the therapeutic relationship between clinician and BPD patient that makes clinicians respond negatively to BPD patients?' These questions have been analyzed both in terms of the emotional and interpersonal difficulties that BPD patients exhibit and in terms of transference/counter-transference relations between clinician and patient. My contribution, instead, is to probe the concepts and values that underlie and shape perception and judgment; here is where conceptual analysis and moral psychology come together. Are clinicians correct in assuming that what I call 'big anger' expressed by patients diagnosed with BPD is symptomatic? But, then, why do many clinicians blame their patients for becoming unreasonably angry? To what extent do assumptions about 'the difficult BPD patient' interfere with empathy and other moral qualities crucial to good therapy? What would it look like to be empathetic when treating BPD patients? This book is a sustained argument that preconceived ideas about BPD patients' impede ethical and therapeutic interactions. Not only empathy is affected; when patients sense a lack of empathy for their distress, they are likely to become more distrustful and, hence, more difficult for clinicians to work with. How can clinicians be trustworthy in this context? These are the kinds of questions to which this book seeks answers.

This task is crucially important because our attitudes, beliefs, perceptions, and judgments provide the conceptual schemas through which we interpret others; if our conceptual schemas are distorted or faulty, our understanding of others is also likely to be flawed. In the clinical context, good theory and practice for clinicians must rest on conceptual and perceptual frameworks that conduce to patient healing – or at least managing of distress. In particular, ethical dimensions of therapy are likely to become tangled and skewed without philosophical clarity of the underlying concepts.

Although guidelines for clinicians working with BPD patients have been published (American Psychiatric Association 2001), they cannot provide a sufficiently rich framework for clinicians. Empathetic research is being conducted and published on therapeutic issues in treatment of BPD – most notably by Marsha Linehan, Mary Zanarini, and John Gunderson – but very little conceptual analysis is performed on the underlying concepts. This is true especially regarding the ethical underpinnings of therapeutic treatment. Therapeutic and ethical considerations ought not to be considered two independent matters; as clinicians know, therapy that is morally problematic is not a good treatment. It is crucial that conceptual, clinical, and ethical questions be brought together when considering what constitutes 'good treatment' for BPD patients. That this project is also clinically informed (see Section iv) suggests that it will be a valuable and unique contribution to the interdisciplinary fields of psychiatry and philosophy.

The primary objective of this book is twofold. First, I aim to provide a rich and nuanced philosophical analysis of some of the central concepts underlying BPD. Second, the point of this exploration is to enhance clinicians' ability to treat patients who exhibit symptoms of BPD in an ethical manner. I expect that an additional contribution to the achievement of these goals will be a clearer understanding of the role that cultural ideas and values about gender do or do not play in diagnosis and treatment of BPD.

As I stated above, analysis is needed because the diagnosis and treatment of BPD rest on a number of concepts that are not clearly understood. Particularly, interesting are the issues of identity disturbance, anger, interpersonal difficulties, impulsivity, self-injury, and manipulativity, all of which are under-analyzed from a philosophical perspective in relation to BPD. A rigorous examination of these issues will provide valuable insight.

Furthermore, women are far more likely to be diagnosed with BPD than are men (Jimenez 1997); in fact, the DSM-IV-TR (2000) reports that 75% of those diagnosed with BPD are women. Mary Ann Jimenez, who has analyzed the psychiatric literature for its evolving thoughts on women, argues that new diagnostic categories continue to reflect a psychiatric orthodoxy where dominant values subjugate women into gender-role conformity (Jimenez 1997; see also Wirth-Couchon (2001) and Becker (1997) both of which authors focus on the BPD diagnosis as it pertains to women). In fact, the picture of the borderline patient as a manipulative, demanding, aggressive, and angry woman is a persistent theme since the diagnosis was included in the DSMs.

The fact that most people diagnosed with BPD are women raises important questions about BPD and gender. Is BPD gendered? If so, in what ways? Are clinicians failing to observe behavior in males that is symptomatic of BPD in females? Men are more likely to be diagnosed with antisocial personality disorder, which in fact raises similar questions about gender and behavior. While the focus of this project is on BPD, it probes assumptions about perceptions of gender, gendered evaluations of behavior, and the impact of social roles on clinical interactions that provide fodder for future researchers interested in patients diagnosed with antisocial personality disorder.

My interest is, ultimately, ethical: What constitutes ethical responses to, and interactions with, someone whom we take to be exhibiting symptoms of BPD? In order to build an ethical framework, I believe it is necessary first to probe from a philosophical perspective those behaviors considered as diagnostic indicators of BPD. As it turns out, the philosophical analysis is enlightening in its own right and not only for its contribution to psychiatric ethics for BPD patients.

(iii) **Flourishing and suffering**

Embedded in this philosophical analysis is the value of flourishing and what it takes not only to flourish ourselves but also to help others flourish to the extent possible. I take a loosely Aristotelian line about flourishing – that it requires that basic material needs to be met, that we need to develop virtues, that we need friends both to be loved and to love, as well as to help us stay virtuous, that we need to be able to make correct inferences (i.e., to reason well), and that we need to have a healthy dose of good luck.

A virtue is a state in which a person feels good, makes decisions, and acts rightly according to what the situation calls for. Virtues are essential for living a fully flourishing life. Virtues of character such as friendship, justice, trustworthiness, industriousness, and integrity enrich us personally and help us live with others cooperatively. Flourishing is an ideal; most of us fall wildly short of it, not only in part because of bad luck, genetics, dysfunctional childhoods and whatnot, but also in part because of poor choices, poor vision, and little impetus to be self-examining and critically conscious.

Mental health is a central condition of flourishing; if our mental stability goes, other areas of our lives become much more difficult. Many mentally ill people can become better able to care for themselves, interact with others, experience a degree of serenity, and feel hopeful. Psychopharmacological developments have been instrumental in the successful treatment of many psychiatric conditions such as schizophrenia and bipolar disorder. Therapeutic treatment is also helpful for many people who suffer from mental illness. The aim of psychiatric treatment both medical and psychological is to restore some autonomy, self-worth, and humanity to the mentally ill. When thinking about flourishing, then, I am including the need for clinicians to grow in virtue and self-reflection so as better to work with their BPD patients and bring them a degree of flourishing in their lives.

(iv) **Methodology**

Philosophical research is conducted in a manner quite different from that of the sciences. By its nature, philosophical investigations are reading intensive.

Following the study of an area of concentration, philosophers do two things: we rigorously examine the terms and concepts employed, and we logically analyze arguments and evaluate them according to longstanding criteria of soundness and validity.

Philosophers typically analyze terms that appear in research and in other scholars' arguments. The aim is to come to a clearer understanding of how a concept is being employed, whether the meaning of the term is held constant in a particular body of literature, and whether the meaning of the term is consistent with meaning and usage across similar domains. A standard way to clarify a concept or term is to identify necessary and sufficient conditions for its usage and definitional status. Understanding of concepts goes beyond dictionary definitions to deeper meanings, often reaching an 'essence' of a concept. In looking for an essence, the aim is to identify those characteristics that make it what it is and not anything else. That is, the objective is to determine what it is that makes a thing *that* thing and nothing else.

While I am wary of using definitions that imply an essence, I do work toward distilling the sense and meaning of a concept. For example, the meaning of 'manipulative' as in 'manipulative behavior' varies not only from the clinical setting to the public setting, but also varies widely within the clinical domain. While listeners and readers may believe that they understand how the concept is being employed and what sort of behaviors are being referred to, the speaker or writer, in reality, may mean a number of different things. The task of a philosopher is to see if all of the meanings that currently fall under the heading of 'manipulativity,' or some other concept, have a commonality. If some of the meanings are better understood as falling within other categories of evaluation, then a philosopher can clarify where distinctions ought to be drawn.

The other aspect of philosophical methodology is the analysis of arguments according to standards of validity and soundness. A valid argument is concerned with the form: How do the premises and conclusions relate to one another? Is the relation a logical one? A valid argument is one where, if all the premises are true, the conclusion must follow. Validity, therefore, allows for false premises. For an argument to be sound, on the other hand, it must meet two conditions: it must be valid and all the premises must be true. The aim of argumentation in philosophical research is to produce sound arguments. These criteria ensure that arguments rest on factual premises and are connected by logical inferences such that the conclusion is warranted. Sound arguments are ones with which any reasoning person assessed of the facts would be able to concur and thus are not merely matters of opinion.

Most arguments do not completely satisfy the conditions for soundness but are nevertheless fairly compelling. The task of a philosopher is not merely to detect which arguments are unsound and to advise rejection of them, but to identify strengths and weaknesses within valid arguments and to sort valid arguments from fallacious ones. The key to doing this evaluation is in identifying missing premises, or assumptions, that would be necessary for an argument to go through but which must themselves be subject to inquiry. In evaluating the reasoning found in the clinical literature, I have closely examined arguments for unstated assumptions, drawing them out and exploring implications of those assumptions for the stated argument and for clinical practice. But readers will find not only the reporting of my analyses of concepts and others' arguments, but also the development of my own arguments. Again, the aim was to construct arguments whose conclusions are persuasive or to open up avenues of inquiry that are suggestive.

I followed the prevailing analytic philosophical approach, with the added component of doing philosophical field work. The idea of philosophical field work was first urged by philosopher J.L. Austin (1956) and is a cornerstone of researcher K.W.M. Fulford (2001). This approach involves a combination of philosophical analysis with an examination of ordinary language uses in everyday contexts (cf. Columbo *et al.*, 2003). Because this approach combines theory with everyday concepts in usage, it is vital to do when conducting responsible philosophical research. For instance, to use the example of 'manipulativity' again, this term frequently is applied to BPD patients, and I offer both a critique of current usage and a distilled and clearer definition of manipulativity. And how does manipulative behavior present itself in an actual clinical interaction? What behavior is the clinician perceiving that he or she is calling 'manipulative'? By observing clinician/patient interactions, I have been able to draw upon clinical experiences as a 'lab' to evaluate my philosophical ideas. Ordinary usage of 'anger' is another example; my critical analysis of the idea of 'too much anger' was checked against actual cases where I saw clinicians sometimes struggling to calm or subdue a patient, only to see the patient's anger escalate. Was this display of anger is the same kind of thing we are thinking of when we grapple with cultural norms that belittle or ignore women's anger and, thus, we try to defend women's anger as (sometimes) legitimate?

Related to the issues of language usage, and at least as important to my project, has been the experience of working with the mentally ill. As I said in the beginning of the introduction, I worked as a certified Crisis Counselor in a seven-county metropolitan area for 5 years (where many clients were assumed to be 'borderline'), and so I have experience with mentally ill patients, emergency rooms, and crisis management. I have worked with sex offenders in the prison system and, while writing this book, I have served as a member of the treatment team for an emergency psychiatric service once a week. I also sit in on therapy sessions as an observer when a psychiatrist with whom I work in EPS meets with a BPD patient. My aim has been to gain first-hand understanding so that my writing is practically informed and sensitive to concrete and actual lived experiences of both patients and clinicians. The clinical observation in my background made it possible for me to integrate my own experiences as a counselor with philosophical thinking and clinicians' expertise – something that I have been doing for several years now. Ethical frameworks for responding to anger have been checked against more practical considerations that arose in the moment between clinician and patient, such as the need to place a patient in restraints. With only a background of the reading literature and thinking about gendered norms for anger, I was skeptical that BPD patients really exhibited out-of-control rage and physical aggression. Clinical experience changed my mind about patient anger (to some extent; see Chapter 2.) These hands-on experiences (so to speak) give me a grounding that provides me with a degree of expertise unusual in a philosopher.

Finally, whenever possible, I bring in patients' voices about their experiences with symptoms associated with BPD and their reactions to the diagnosis itself. As Nadine Nehls has learned from research into patients' perspectives, 'to learn from a person with mental health problems is to challenge the reification and stigmatization of any classification system' (Nehls 1999, p. 291; cf. also Fallon 2003). One thing that some patients tell us is that, while they believe that the criteria fit, they see no benefit to having the diagnosis when it comes to treatment (Nehls 1999, p. 288.) Other patients raise questions about the fitness of certain criteria such as identity disturbance (Miller 1994). Sadly, little material is available from BPD patients' perspectives.[2] But what literature and research exist can bring life, realism, and particularity to otherwise abstract discussion.

(v) The structure of the book

This book is divided into two parts. Part I, which includes Chapters 1 through 6, pursues the philosophical investigation of concepts and issues in the diagnosis and treatment of BPD. The issues analyzed are identity disturbance, excessive anger, unstable interpersonal relationships, impulsivity, self-injury, and manipulativity. Each chapter includes examples and is informed by my clinical observations and experience, as well as by the clinical, philosophical, sociological, and anthropological literature when relevant. Part II, consisting of Chapters 7 through 9, presents a theoretical framework for ethically responsible diagnosis and treatment based on insights gleaned from Part I as well as clinical observations. I first provide a general framework for ethics that takes into account the discoveries and understandings from Part I. The theory of

---

[2] The exception is found on Internet sites. However, these sites are set up for BPD patients and their families, and I believe it is a violation of the honor system for me to listen in on them for research purposes without IRB approval and all that that entails.

ethics that I use is virtue ethics and, in Chapter 7, I explain why I focus on virtue. Part II discusses three specific virtues that I take to be especially important in working with BPD patients. The first virtue is 'trustworthiness,' a virtue that is the corollary of being trusted. Many BPD patients are deeply distrustful of others, even when those others are, objectively, trustworthy. I set out features of trustworthiness and explain how and why clinicians need to cultivate trustworthiness with respect to their patients. The second virtue I discuss is called 'giving uptake' and is a conversational and listening form of the interaction that I spell out in Chapter 8. The third virtue is empathy. In Chapter 9, I say why it is important to think of empathy as a virtue and why it is absolutely crucial that clinicians develop empathy with their BPD patients. In this chapter, though, I also take up ontological questions about the status of BPD as a mental disorder – questions that have been lurking throughout.

(vi) **What this book is not**

This book is admittedly ambitious, but a few caveats are in order. First of all, I have left out any historical discussion of how BPD came into being; readers interested in that background should see Gunderson and Links (2008, Ch. 1) and Kroll (1988, Ch. 1). Secondly, I do not include the recent studies that examine possible links between BPD and brain sciences; although that is a fruitful and crucial area of research, it is a relatively new field of study and the normative questions I raise here are likely still to be relevant for quite some time. Thirdly, this book isn't meant to be a handbook on how to do therapy. It is true that I focus on ethico-therapeutic issues in working with BPD patients, but my aim is to urge clinicians to be critically self-reflective about the background assumptions, norms, expectations, and so on, that undergird this diagnosis. Such effort, I believe, will be rewarded by more positive and, thus, more effective therapy in the long run, but readers who work as clinicians will need to rely on the body of information available to them about doing therapy with BPD patients. Finally, and most important for me to say: I am not offering a definitive analysis of BPD; I am not taking a position on debates about the categorical versus dimensional model; I am not presenting the best extant definitions of what a mental disorder is; and I am not arguing that BPD does or does not fall under that definition. Instead, I analyze what I take to be particularly messy and confused constructs that underlie this diagnosis. The conclusions I draw along the way may add up to an overhaul of the diagnosis, but I leave that decision to others. For my part, I will be pleased if this book prompts vigorous discussion and moral and epistemic engagement about and with the population saddled with the diagnosis of BPD.

(vii) **Acknowledgements**

It's hard to know where to start in thanking those who've been instrumental in bringing this book forth. I'm sure to forget people so I apologize in advance. And in a sense, I've been working on this diagnosis and the people affected by it for 20 years now, ever since I began work as a crisis counselor. That's a long time for anyone to remember all the people who've helped them along the way. But certainly, I want to thank Douglas Lewis, Michael Root, and Naomi Scheman for working with me on an early paper on BPD while I was in graduate school. I am indebted to Norman Dahl for many aspects of my intellectual education but, especially, for first handing me a Call for Papers on recovered memories for an organization I hadn't known about – the Association for the Advancement of Philosophy and Psychiatry (AAPP) – where I presented my first work in philosophy and psychiatry and met John Sadler and other AAPP folks; Norman as well as Naomi Scheman nurtured my early interest in bringing together philosophy and psychiatry and I am forever grateful to them for that. John Sadler, M.D., has encouraged me from the day we first met (at that AAPP conference on recovered memories) and who has read numerous versions of chapters and, in philosophy and psychiatry in general, has surely devoted more time to my interdisciplinary writing than anyone could expect. Jerome Kroll, M.D., also has read much of this book in its various permutations and has kept me on my toes; I am fortunate that he has the clinical and scholarly background in BPD by which to guide me (although I wasn't always willing to be guided). Bill Fulford, Jennifer Radden, and Peter Zachar have read parts of the book and have questioned me, challenged me, and sharpened my thinking; Peter's and my work on PDs as medical and moral kinds has enhanced greatly my appreciation of BPD as a messy kind of thing. The faculty of the Institute for Bioethics, Health Policy, and Law in Louisville, and the AAPP Executive Council members have patiently (at least in appearance) listened not only to the content of my arguments but also to my frustrations and anxieties as this work progressed (or didn't). Robert Kimball did all of this and more: he tolerated my long writing spurts, sympathized with my 'I just can't write' days, hailed my ambitions about this book, and soothed my neurotic tendencies. He even occasionally would take what was supposed to be my turn grocery shopping – a kindness I tried not to exploit. My family, as it is loosely construed, has been wonderfully supportive about this project over the years as I have taken up valuable fun time with talking about the questions and problems that have consumed me. Andrea Sinclair has worked diligently as my research assistant – meaning that she did the tiresome part of writing a book – word-by-word editing, and Carol Maxwell has guided me well (and gently) through the publication process.

I can't imagine being able to write this book without the clinical experience I have been granted here in Louisville. I am grateful to Allan Tasman, M.D., for opening doors for me; Steve Lippman, M.D., for allowing me to shadow him in the in-patient ward; Gordon Strauss, M.D., for allowing me to observe him at Emergency Psychiatric Services (EPS); and Rifaat El-Mallakh, M.D., who invited me in, included me, and mentored me more than I can express (thank you Rif). Warm thanks to the entire crew at EPS, who answered my incessant questions and allowed me to imagine myself useful to the treatment team.

Finally, my respect and gratitude go to all the patients who were willing to let me learn from them. There is no substitute for real people when trying to learn. May this book help you and your loved ones.

Part I

Chapter 1

Identity disturbance and the self

1.1 Statement of the problem

One of the criteria for diagnosing borderline personality disorder (BPD) is identity disturbance. Identity disturbances include such things as feelings of emptiness or unintegrated and contradictory self-images (Gunderson 2001; Goldstein 1995). Interestingly, though, the clinical literature offers little in the way of understanding identity disturbance, or even what the constructs of 'identity' and 'identity disturbance' are. As Tess Wilkinson-Ryan and Drew Westen say, the literature variously refers to BPD identity confusion as 'fragmentation, boundary confusion, and lack of cohesion... These concepts are difficult to operationalize, however, and several questions remain, such as the extent to which identity disturbance is a unitary phenomenon ...' (Wilkinson-Ryan and Westen 2000, p. 528). Theodore Millon describes identity crises as 'nebulous symptom clusters' (Millon 1996, p. 205). Furthermore, little research is directed at understanding identity disturbance in BPD patients. One notable exception is the work of Zanarini *et al.* (1998), who examined dysphoric states reported by patients diagnosed with BPD. One cluster of characteristics came under the construct of 'identitylessness,' which included 'feeling like I am evil, like a small child, unreal, like people and things aren't real, like people can see right through me, like I have no identity, like I'm someone else, like other people are living inside me' (Zanarini *et al.* 1998, p. 205). These researchers report that, along with other states, identitylessness, understood as an 'absence of a core feeling of continuity about oneself,' contributes to 'despair and desperation among borderline patients that may not be appreciated by even the most knowledgeable of clinicians' (p. 205). However, Sharon Miller suggests that BPD women view themselves as estranged from others and inadequate according to social standards but not as having an impaired sense of self or an identity disturbance (Miller 1994).

This chapter raises questions about the construct of identity that is prevalent in Western psychiatry – that is, a construct that neglects the impact of an increasingly obsessive interest in acquisitiveness and consumerism in producing feelings of emptiness; that neglects the subordinate status of females in medicalizing identity confusion; and that assumes that where boundaries between 'inner' and 'outer' are drawn is universal across cultures. The effects of materialism, and gender and cultural differences, press against the prevailing view of identity disturbance. There are elements in each of these factors that challenge the prevailing view – factors that have an impact on interpreting women who fit the diagnosis of BPD – and this chapter develops these themes below. We diagnose through symptoms, so it is crucial that we examine both those cultural pressures and influences and the way we come to see certain behaviors as symptoms. This chapter, then, takes issue with the values that underlie the metaphysics of self-identity as it pertains to mental health. Yet experiences of identity problems can be troublesome and distressing for the patient. Such experiences can disrupt her interpersonal relationships and exacerbate a sense of alienation from others, prompting other behaviors such as impulsivity or self-injury in order temporarily to fill the void. Clinicians cannot ignore patients' expressions of identity issues regardless of the messiness and assumptions of the concept.

1.2 **The Western construct**

Self-identity is at the heart of Western conceptions of the healthy human subject. The normative modern self, in the philosophical and psychiatric literature, is unified, stable, and individuated from others while maintaining stable and healthy relationships with others. Those who do not experience themselves this way, or are not perceived by others this way, are viewed as mentally unhealthy. The Western construct of identity in the clinical literature, summarized by Tess Wilkinson-Ryan and Drew Westen, who drew on extensive literature reviews, is characterized as follows:

> a sense of continuity over time; emotional commitment to a set of self-defining representations of self, role relationships, and core values and ideal self-standards; development or acceptance of a world view that gives life meaning; and some recognition of one's place in the world by significant others.

> (Wilkinson-Ryan and Westen 2000, p. 529)

'Having' self-identity, though, also requires that one is aware of being unified, etc. Identity, thus, is a self-aware sense of oneself as a distinct being who holds commitments and values that are to some degree self-defining, who is relatively consistent in those values over time, and who is able emotionally to connect with others in a stable manner. Identity thus has both internal components (in terms of mental representations of self and other) and external ones (in terms of interpersonal relations, the expression of emotions, the articulation of commitments, and so on).

Therefore, the construct of identity occurs within a system of representations that not only includes identity but also selfhood, personhood, and self-awareness (Neisser 1997). And systems of representations are never universals; they are embedded in particular historical moments and within cultures and practices. What is included in a system of representations, and what work it is supposed to do, varies widely (cf. Kay 2000, Ch. 1). So, how do historical and cultural contingencies affect the particular mode of representation that is identity?

1.3 **Boundaries**

Philosophical meanings of the term 'identity' range from identity as in $x = x$ to social, to ethnic, to personal identity and many in between. The meaning of identity that is relevant to this analysis is identity as a sense of self, where our personal identity typically is informed by social, religious, ethnic, sexual, gender, and role identity. Identity as a sense of self is a fairly recent construct that arose in the West in tandem with that of the individual who has rights and duties. With the rise of individual rights, the need developed for distinct boundaries to identify individuals. Important to my discussion, therefore, is the notion that identity is something bounded and that what is contained within those boundaries is normative. So let me talk about boundaries a bit.

1.3.1 **Why boundaries are thought to be important to identity**

Boundaries are conceptual constructs that provide figures of thought and allow us to perform mental operations and construct categories (Barth 2000, pp. 17 and 19). They allow us to make discriminations among and between objects and ideas, thus making it possible for us to order the world. This way of thinking about objects and boundaries draws on Western philosophical and psychodynamic theories of the self. Objects can be constructs like 'desk' or 'woman' but they can also be people with whom the young child most closely interacts. Philosophers ranging from Aristotle to Kant have long argued that, in order to think at all, we must sort things into categories and kinds. Jean Piaget's research shows the stages of mastery by which a child's cognition logically develops and progresses toward intellectual maturity (cf. Piaget 1999). In psychodynamic theory, the idea is that by recognizing the caregiver(s) as discrete, bounded objects, the child introjects them (takes them into his psychic world) as internal mental representations. Object-relations theorists such as Otto Kernberg theorize that bounded objects are organized as 'relatively stable configurations of mental processes' (Kernberg 1984, p. 4; see also

Gabbard (2001) for an overview of BPD and psychodynamic theories). This structural organization is what stabilizes the mental world and shapes the structure of personality. A flawed psychic structural organization and poor quality of internal objects are said to form the symptoms of BPD. And, as the chapters in Part I will suggest, BPD patients may make cognitive mistakes in discriminating, categorizing, and reasoning about themselves and others that are associated with their distress, for example, by the primitive defense mechanism of splitting.

Millon argues that structural disorganization is the *sine qua non* of personality disorders (1996, pp. 609–613; cf. Introduction on definitions of personality and personality disorder). In particular, splitting can be understood as a mistake in the content of object boundaries. Splitting is an unconscious process of dividing external objects into 'good' and 'bad.' It can also include oscillating between 'good' and 'bad' self-concepts. In splitting, the boundaries drawn between 'good' and 'bad' people are rigid; the categories are held as mutually exclusive and admit no overlap or integration between the two. The result is a sense of oneself as inadequate, evil, or empty alternating with grandiosity and entitlement, and a perception of others as all good or all bad. When splitting becomes entrenched in a person's personality structure, it can be very difficult for that person to feel fulfilled and to have fulfilling relationships with others. Whether or not that structural organization is rightly called identity, it makes sense that not just any way of internally ordering a culture's foundational concepts and object relations will do. Note that, because early childhood experience is usually considered to be at least part of the etiology of damaged structural organization of the personality, it would be inaccurate to say that such mistakes in perception and belief are solely the result of poor cognitive skills. But difficulties with anger, impulsivity, relationships, and so on may partly be the result of flawed reasoning, such as considering someone as untrustworthy who hasn't merited distrust or engaging in repeated unsafe casual sex without considering the potentially harmful consequences to oneself.

This way of thinking about identity allows us to begin to understand what is distressing when something goes awry. Rigid, dichotomous thinking about others and contradictory and oscillating self-identity are typical of BPD patients (cf. Linehan 1993, esp. Ch. 1). Fear, anger, desperation, and anxiety may be expressions of the distress of poor-quality internal objects and problematic personality structure. The reason for this distress might be seen in terms of a fundamental need in the animal kingdom for beings to form internal attachment objects that can sooth and reassure when the environment is perceived as threatening. In normal healthy development, the maturing child learns to hold mental representations of self-object and of others that are 'good enough' to present the world as a safe place and, in the temporary absence of concrete loving others, to soothe oneself. Without such internal representations of self and other, the developing person searches for external objects (persons, experiences, events) that can serve as substitutes.

Sander Gilman (1985) situates these issues of identity in psycho-political terms. To avoid confronting the contradictions of 'good' and 'bad' within ourselves and to maintain a sense of control over the world, we project the 'bad' onto some others. The boundary between self and other is an illusion, though. 'Because there is no real line between self and other, an imaginary line must be drawn; and so that the illusion of an absolute difference between self and other is never troubled, this line is as dynamic in its ability to alter itself as is the self' (Gilman 1985, p. 18). Gilman argues that stereotypes function to preserve the boundary between self and other when self-integration is threatened. Stereotypes allow us to mark the difference between self and other and regain a sense of control. But '[f]or the pathological personality every confrontation sets up this echo' (Gilman 1985, p. 18). While for Gilman, pathology is manifested through racist stereotypes that are entrenched in a person's psyche, for psychiatry, the pathology of BPD identity disturbance is manifested through the oscillation between 'good' self and 'bad' self, 'good other' and 'bad' other,' with little or no ability to integrate evaluations and accept gradations of qualities in oneself and others. When splitting or stereotyping is so entrenched that reason and evidence cannot override them, then we have a problem.

1.3.2 Boundaries and cultural differences

I agree with the prevailing view that boundaries between self and other, between inner and outer self, and between good and bad are constructs that provide a sense of control over our world. The structural organization of constructs and categories as well as the content of those categories form the basis of our interactions and ways of being in the world. But, although people typically have a sense of themselves as being bounded, their accounts of what constitutes the bounded identity differ from culture to culture. Anthropologist Clifford Geertz stated back in 1975 that:

> ... the Western conception of the person as a bounded, unique, more or less integrated motivational and cognitive universe, a dynamic center of awareness, emotion, judgment, and action organized into a distinctive whole and set contrastively both against other such wholes and against a social and natural background is, however incorrigible it may seem to us, a rather peculiar idea within the context of the world's cultures.

(Geertz 1975, p. 48)

For example, the Baktaman identity seems to be formed by bonds and not boundaries, meaning that identity emphasizes connection and relationality with others more than it emphasizes one's edges, limits, and demarcations of the self (Barth 2000, p. 24), and the Maori world is organized by networks of kinship and alliance, a cosmology of 'nets of relationship between people and places, animated by reciprocal exchanges' described in relational terms (Salmond 2000, p. 52). Disruption of identity in that model results in illness. Norms for a given culture, then, strongly influence where the 'inner' and 'outer' boundaries are drawn and what can and cannot belong 'inside.'

1.4 Boundaries, the self–other relation, and the concept of alterity

As Gilman's work suggests (1985) in order to understand identity, we not only need to think about boundaries, but also about the construct of 'the other' or what is also called 'alterity.' Bruce Janz writes that, 'The other serves the function of making oneself coherent, either by mirroring or by alienating, and serves as the locus of complexity in any narrative of coherence' (Janz 1997, p. 233). Theoretical understandings of the other range from Aristotle's idea of the friend as another self (Aristotle 1985) to Levinas's work (1961), which treats the other as utterly alien. As with categorizing in general – where part of knowing, say, what a chair is involves grasping what it is not – the construction of boundaries of the Western self involves coming to understand who and what we are in terms of who and what we are not. In each case, the domain is specified: 'not-chair' is in terms of things to sit upon (rather than all possible objects other than 'chair') and 'not-self' is in terms of other human beings (rather than all possible objects other than 'self'). In normal, healthy development, the infant is able to individuate and separate from her caregiver such that she comes to see herself as separate from, but connected to, her caregiver. The caregiver is an other, but not an alien other but another self, another subject. Ideally, the ebb and flow of self–other relations will result in intersubjectivity, where two subjects relate to one another by affirming each's subjectivity while maintaining one's own, with just enough fluidity in boundaries to allow for the mirroring of subjectivity in the other.

The self–other relationship is not only psychological but also deeply political. Beauvoir (1972) argues that, under patriarchy, the self/subject is male and the other is female and secondary both in terms of knowledge production and in terms of subjective consciousness. Female consciousness, according to Beauvoir, is subjugated, and hence thwarted in its development and ability to exercise autonomy. Fanon (1982) argues that, under colonialism, the Negro identity is a negation, 'not-white.' Both argue that patterns of identity formation that systematically demote women of all colors and male and female Blacks to inferior others are profoundly damaging and distorting to members of dominated groups.

Nevertheless, the other need not to be thought of as alienating or engulfing. Janz says that 'otherness has many faces' and, because his discussion is so illuminating, I quote it at length:

> *Fascination.* The Other can be the exotic, the foreign. It could be the object of idle curiosity, of collection, and of pride.
>
> *Repulsion.* The Other can be the thing to be avoided, the leper. It could be that which reminds me of my own corrigibility, or that which just turns my stomach.
>
> *Desire.* The Other can be the thing to be owned or controlled. It is that which I believe fulfills a lack in my existence.
>
> *Dependence.* The Other can be the thing which makes my own existence possible. According to Karl Barth and Rudolph Otto (to use an analogy from theology), it is the Otherness of God that is the real point of religion. It could be the ground of my being or it could be the transcendence of my being; either way, it is what I am not, but what makes me possible.
>
> *Smugness.* The Other could be the primitive (Levy–Bruhl), the ones not like us because they lack culture. They could be valorized (Rousseau) or vilified (Hegel); but, they are always easily forgotten.
>
> *Appropriation/subsumption.* The Other could be that which is absorbed, and which is assimilated into my being, giving up its own being on my behalf.
>
> *Marginalization.* The Other is often that which is left out after coherent meaning is arrived at. It is that which makes no sense, from the point of view of the coherent center.
>
> *Horizon.* The Other might be that which holds the possibility of understanding by being the place where tradition and prejudice can be uncovered, at least in part.
>
> *Domination.* The Other could be that which is my servant and that which relieves me from the drudgery of my own existence by taking that drudgery on him-, her-, or itself. The machine and the slave are both the Other.
>
> *Foil.* The Other could be that against which I test myself or that against which I measure myself.
>
> *Mirror.* The Other could be that in which I find myself again and meet myself anew, the familiar in the alien, and the alien in the familiar.
>
> *Body.* The Other could be that part of me that is always subordinate, if I believe Descartes and hold that I am a thinking thing. It may simply reduce to a tool that I can use to control other thinking things, or it could be the thing that keeps me from true Enlightenment (Plato, Gnostics). It could also be that which requires interpretation, as it is my expression in the world and the world's interaction with me (Merleau-Ponty).

(Janz 1997, p. 231–232)

The recognition of many forms of otherness is useful because it moves us away from more simplistic dichotomous thinking that forms the prevailing concept of identity in Western psychiatry, psychology, and popular culture. This is especially the case with respect to the idea of the other as mirror, again as it suggests connection, mutuality, and perhaps mutual intersubjective growth.

A wonderfully rich (if complicated) way of thinking about otherness or alterity comes from Ricoeur, who argues that the self is included in the other in a dialectic. Ricoeur explains:

> A kind of otherness that is not (or not merely) the result of comparison is suggested by our title, otherness of a kind that can be constitutive of self-hood as such. *Oneself as Another* suggests from the outset that the selfhood of oneself implies otherness to such an intimate degree that one cannot be thought of without the other, that instead one passes into the other, as we might say in Hegelian terms.
>
> (Ricoeur 1992, p. 3)[1]

One important consequence of this dialectic is that the (ipse)[2] self does not imply an unchanging character. Ricoeur argues that otherness is constitutive of the self:

> The fact that otherness is not added on to selfhood from outside, as though to prevent its solipsistic drift, but that it belongs instead to the tenor of meaning and to the ontological constitution of selfhood is a feature that strongly distinguishes this third dialectic from that of selfhood and sameness, which maintains a preeminently disjunctive character.
>
> (Ricoeur 1992, p. 317)

The ipse self, on this view, is not foundational, nor is it unified; otherness and self are conjoined 'following a diversity of centers of otherness' (p. 318). For Ricoeur, then, alterity is polysemous and irreducible. As David Vessey explains, 'our identity is never simply our own. It is embedded in relations with others and we do not have ultimate control over the nature of these relationships much less the nature of our identity' (Vessey 2002).

---

1 'To "as" [in *Oneself as Another*] I should like to attach a strong meaning, not only that of a comparison (oneself similar to another) but indeed that of an implication (oneself in as much as being other)' Ricoeur.

2 Ricoeur draws upon a distinction in Latin between idem-identity and ipse-identity; the former is what gives self-sameness in the spatiotemporal domain and the latter is what gives self its uniqueness and the ability to assign intention to oneself. Ricoeur argues that both are necessary and necessarily intertwined in what it means to have an identity.

These ideas turn out to be important in understanding BPD identity disturbance. For, what does the borderline patient do with alterity?[3]

For the BPD patient, the other typically is either held rigidly at bay or is viewed as another to absorb, dominate, or become. Permeable boundaries are experienced as threatening but, at the same time, the desire for recognition from the other and to fill one's emptiness propels the BPD patient into boundary disruptions. Problems with boundaries and alterity, then, trap her in her simultaneous desire for and fear of intimacy. This disruptive aspect of personality structure is said to be a mark of identity disturbance.

1.5 What is 'identity disturbance?'

So far, I have discussed the concept of identity from a Western perspective and have begun to complicate this picture by drawing on Ricoeur's argument that otherness is constitutive of the self. But the aim of this chapter is not only to understand the construct of identity, as it is used in the clinical literature, but also to understand the construct of identity disturbance since the latter forms one of the criteria for the diagnosis of BPD.

I discussed earlier the role that boundaries between self and other play in the formation and maintenance of identity. But identity involves much more than just having appropriate boundaries.

Systematizing the clinical and theoretical literature, Westen and Cohen summarized the major attributes of identity disturbance that are hypothesized to be central to BPD.

> These include a lack of consistently invested goals, values, ideals, and relationships; a tendency to make temporary hyperinvestments in roles, values systems, world views, and relationships that ultimately break down and lead to a sense of emptiness and meaninglessness; gross inconsistencies in behavior over time and across situations that lead to a relatively accurate perception of the self as lacking coherence; difficulty integrating multiple representations of self at any given time; a lack of a coherent life narrative or sense of continuity over time; and a lack of continuity of relationships over time that leaves significant parts of the patient's past 'deposited' with people who are no longer part of the individual's life, and hence the loss of shared memories that help define the self over time.

> (Wilkinson-Ryan and Westen 2000, p. 529)

Wilkinson-Ryan and Westen found that identity issues in BPD patients did not readily map onto theorized components of identity disturbance. Their study of BPD patients identified four factors of identity disturbance. But these factors

---

[3] Thanks to Giovanni Stanghellini for putting this question to me.

were not all equally correlated with identity disturbance: 'painful incoherence was most highly associated with presence of identity disturbance ...' (p. 538).[4] Modestin *et al.* (1998) also examined the construct of identity disturbance. In their study, identity disturbance was 'defined by uncertainty about at least two of the following: self image, sexual orientation, long-term goals or career choice, type of friends desired, and preferred values' (p. 353). But they point out that the typical BPD patient is young and that evidence suggests that this criterion is age dependent (Modestin 1998, p. 352). Millon discusses the symptoms that sometimes appear as a prelude to BPD:

> These youngsters are characterized by vague feelings of apathy and boredom, and inability to see any meaning or purpose to life other than momentary gratifications and an aimless and drifting existence without commitment of direction. These young-sters feel estranged from society's traditions and believe them to be false or deceiving, but are unable or unwilling to find an alternative to replace them.
>
> (Millon 1996, p. 666)

But uncertainty about self-image, choice of friends, and other life issues is commonplace among adolescents. And adolescent girls have an especially difficult time – at least in American life – sorting out what kind of women they want to become. As Lyn Mikel Brown and Carol Gilligan write, 'Girls at this time have been observed to lose their vitality, their resilience, their immunity to depression, their sense of themselves and their character' (1992, p. 2). Brown and Gilligan's findings suggest that adolescence for girls is a time of confusion, loss of voice, inner division, and difficulty staying connected with others.

Cathy Leaker, herself diagnosed as borderline, describes the problem that arises with the notion of identity disturbance:

> The borderline is persistently figured as an individual unable to make stable and con-sistent, and therefore appropriate and responsible, choices: three of the nine criteria listed in the DSM-IV address this fundamental deficiency. Of course, these criteria are not 'explained' in terms of choice (because most of us, given the heritage of humanist individualism, value choice far too much to pathologize it) but rather as, to quote directly from Criterion 3, 'markedly and persistently unstable sense of self ' (American Psychiatric Association, 1994, p. 654). Criterion 3 is further explained in the DSM text as 'sudden and dramatic shifts in self-image, characterized by shifting goals, values, and vocational aspirations' (p. 651). It seems at least possible to me given the particular examples listed—career, sexual identity, values, and types of friends (p. 651)—that one

---

4 The four factors were role absorption, in which patients appeared to absorb themselves in, or define themselves in terms of, a specific role, cause, or unusual group. The second factor, painful incoherence, reflected patients' subjective experience and concern about a lack of coherence. The third factor, inconsistency, was characterized less by subjective than objective incoherence (i.e., did not imply distress). The fourth factor was lack of commitment (i.e. to jobs or values) (Wilkinson-Ryan and Westen 2000, p. 535).

man's identity disturbance is another woman's 'consciousness-raising,' her right not only to choose but to make multiple choices in response to her culture, personal development, and life situation.

(Leaker 2002, pp. 245–146)

I think Leaker is right when she argues that responsible diagnosis of BPD patients requires that their voices be taken into account, and she suggests that the notion of identity disturbance is ideologically linked to an historically and culturally situated construct of identity. Furthermore, Leaker points to a potential gender bias in evaluating uncertainty and emptiness as a symptom of pathology. Girls have a harder time of feeling part of a larger community and society without experiencing painful double-binds, contradictory demands, and the threat of not being recognized and valued as a subject: women's social position as a class is that of the other (Beauvoir 1972). To better understand those who present with symptoms of BPD, then, we need not only to examine the science of personality disorders but culturally-inflected beliefs and values as well.

1.6 **Problems with the constructs**

Millon takes the view that some aspects of normalcy are universal and therefore culture-free. Normalcy, on his view, is characterized by the 'capacity to function autonomously and competently, a tendency to adjust to one's social milieu effectively and efficiently, a subjective sense of contentment and satisfaction, and the ability to self-actualize or to fulfill one's potentials' (Millon 1996, p. 13). Although he acknowledges that historical and cultural factors may affect what constitutes normalcy, he also says that the borderline personality has 'a *very* small probability of falling at the normal end of the continuum in almost all cultures' (p. 13, emphasis in original).

Nevertheless, there are three reasons to examine the equation of identity with psychological health and of identity disturbances with mental disorder.

First, emptiness and a feeling that life is meaningless is a phenomenon that, arguably, has become increasingly common and problematic in the past 50 years. I consider the possibility that shifts in Western culture, particularly in increasing materialism, produce emptiness and alienation. If this hypothesis is right, the task is to understand why some people become particularly distressed and anguished while others find ways to mask or fill their emptiness to prevent debilitating suffering. The second reason to analyze the values underpinning the concept of self-identity concerns gender. As a class, girl children and women of all ethnic groups experience subordination, disrespect, invisibility, and other forms of oppression – even in societies that have increasingly offered females more opportunities for development and free choices (Brettell and Sargent 1993). It is not surprising that the mixed messages and the thwarted attempts to actualize their goals may create, in some women, feelings of emptiness and contradictory senses of the self. I raise the question whether emptiness and uncertainty, in this context, should be viewed as a symptom of a mental disorder. The third reason to examine the prevailing concept of identity is related to its place holder as a manifestation of dominating forms of identity formation and social organization. Cross-cultural studies indicate that many cultures have quite a different way of drawing the boundaries between the inner self and the external world. I therefore consider arguments that the conception of identity as unified is a product of dominant Western cultures.

1.6.1 **Materialism and emptiness**

Philip Cushman (1990) argues that the unquestioned assumption of self-contained individualism in psychology is ethnocentric (p. 599). The charge of ethnocentrism is important because ethnocentrism is culturally disrespectful and acts as a form of psychological imperialism. Cushman's articulation of the self is useful:

> The self embodies what the culture believes is humankind's place in the cosmos: its limits, talents, expectations, and prohibitions. In this sense the self is an aspect of what Heidegger called the horizon of shared understandings or 'the clearing' carved out by the particular practices of a particular culture. There is no universal, transhistorical self, only local selves; no universal theory about the self, only local theories.
>
> (Cushman 1990, p. 599)

According to Cushman, the current Western conception of the self as bounded and masterful is empty. 'By this I mean that our terrain has shaped a self that experiences a significant absence of community, tradition, and shared meaning. It experiences these social absences and their consequences "interiorly" as a lack of personal conviction and worth, and it embodies the absences as a chronic, undifferentiated emotional hunger' (Cushman 1990, p. 600). The role of the state is to provide the illusion and the means for people temporarily to fill themselves up and experience cohesion. This is done through an economy that [emphasizes] spending money and the motivation to continue doing so (p. 601). But '[psychiatry] has continued to decontextualize the individual, examining the patient as an isolated entity without considering the larger sociohistorical causes of personal distress. As a result, cultural absences and political wounds are "interiorized" (i.e. located in the self) ...' (Cushman 1990, p. 609). On this view, people experience emptiness because the emphasis on individualism and the flawed concept of identity give rise to a hunger for community, relationship, and meaningfulness that cannot be satisfied except temporarily and in superficial ways.

Notice how similar Cushman's account of materialist emptiness is to the psychiatric construct of identity disturbance:

> Inner emptiness may be expressed in many ways, such as low self-esteem (the absence of a sense of personal worth), values confusion (the absence of a sense of personal convictions), eating disorders (the compulsion to fill the emptiness with food, or to embody the emptiness by refusing food), drug abuse (the compulsion to fill the emptiness with chemically induced emotional experiences), and chronic consumerism (the compulsion to fill the emptiness with consumer items and the experience of 'receiving' something from the world. It may also take the form of an absence of personal meaning.

(Cushman 1990, p. 604)

Yet Cushman locates the problem in sociohistorical and cultural shifts that are specific to Western modernization and economies and not as universal dysfunctions in a particular population with a personality disorder. Cushman argues that a common sales strategy for promoting products is that of promising the buyer a new identity if she purchases that product (Cushman 1990, p. 605). This is especially true for women; advertising and marketing create inadequacy in order to promote sales. American culture, in particular, promulgates hunger, envy, and greed in individuals such that those feelings deeply influence our motivations, felt needs, and sense of ourselves (Wachtel 2003, pp. 104–106). The borderline symptoms of emotional hunger and possessiveness, and rage or depression when those needs are thwarted thus can be understood to occur in a culture of greed and acquisitiveness.

1.6.2 The female gender and emptiness

Social identity theorists emphasize the idea that how we view ourselves is deeply influenced by how others evaluate and treat us. An understanding of sex and gender as stimulus variables helps to shift the study of identity from something ahistorical and static to something influenced by the expectations, values, and attitudes males hold toward females. The prevailing view of the mature, psychologically healthy, and morally responsible person has been male, and critics have come to dub this normative view *the autonomous man* (cf. Code 1991). Autonomy, say the critics, is assumed to correlate positively with rationality and objectivity, traits that females are taken to be deficient in. Science, conceived as quintessentially objectivist, is driven by the metaphysics of the person as 'essentially solitary, separate, self-subsistent beings, fundamentally opaque to one another' (Code 1991, p. 52). Thus, gendered norms of identity intersect with those of autonomy and choice to produce value-laden notions of freedom, subjectivity, and agency, as Lorraine Code argues:

> Consider autonomy. Its construction and valuation as a masculine character trait either effaces the very possibility of female autonomy or asserts that the autonomy women achieve is of different worth. Jane Martin observes that 'when a woman displays … rationality and autonomy … she is derided for what are considered negative, unpleasant characteristics, even as her male colleagues are admired for possessing them' Autonomy and rationality are not the gender-neutral traits many philosophers have assumed.
>
> (Code 1991, p. 120)

If the critics of the traditional view of autonomy are correct, they lend support to Leaker's skepticism about the possibility that identity disturbance is scientifically legitimate.

Challenges to the autonomous man model within the clinical fields of psychiatry and psychology began in the early 1980s when Carol Gilligan and others argued for a construct of identity that is relational (1982). (These challenges had been around for decades in philosophy but had not reached these other disciplines). Gilligan not only proposed this construct as a theory by which we could better understand identity but also as an empirical claim about gendered differences in self-conception and experiences of the self–other relationship. (I return to these claims in Chapter 3). The relational model would seem to suggest that the norms of unity, self-continuity, and boundedness are more likely to produce mental distress. What occurs when a culture holds both models but equates each with a gender and promulgates gender inequities? It is not surprising that many girls and women are expressing confusion, uncertainty, and fragmentation.

1.6.3 Culture

Cultural psychiatry raises questions about whether or not the assumed 'basic concepts' of psychology such as person, identity, representation, knowledge activation, and information-seeking are in fact 'basic.' As Kathryn Linn Geurts says, 'While not denying that there may be certain psychic universals within the human species, cultural psychologists argue that "psychologists may be prematurely settling on *one* psychology, that is on one set of assumptions about what are the relevant or most important psychological states and processes, and on one set of generalizations about their nature and function"' (Geurts 2002, p. 15, quoting Markus, Kitayama, and Heiman; emphasis in original). As Cushman says, 'culture "completes" humans by explaining and interpreting the world, helping them to focus their attention on or ignore certain aspects of their environment, and instructing and forbidding them to think and act in certain ways' (Cushman 1990, p. 601). Similarly, Gyekye

(1987) and Mudimbe (1988) argue that 'identity issues cannot be understood without archaeologies of specific (African) modes of philosophy and thought' (Geurts 2002, p. 171).

To that end, I offer as an example a discussion of the work of Kathryn Geurts. Geurts studied the sensorium (sensory order) of Anlo-Ewe people of Western Africa. Her reason for this study is that 'a culture's sensory order is one of the first and most basic elements of making ourselves human' and that the moods and dispositions that the sensoriums are built upon 'become fundamental to an expectation of what it is to be a person in a given time and place' (2002, p. 5). The senses, according to Geurts, are 'ways of embodying cultural categories' that 'constitute vital aspects of a people's sense of identity, and within the notion of identity, I believe, are subsumed their ideas and experiences of well-being and their conceptions of the person and the self' (p. 10). Drawing upon the work of Thomas Csordas, she argues that self-processes, rather than self as an independent entity, engage us in culture so that cultural motifs are thematized in ways that allow for a culturally constituted 'identity' to emerge (p. 237). The Anlo-Ewe have a term called 'seselelame,' meaning something like 'feel-feel at flesh inside,' an expression which highlights a whole-body sensory awareness that is at once a bodily way of knowing what is happening to you and an internal sense of balance. As I understand it, balance is both a sense and a skill that one draws upon in learning to hear within the body so as to move in culturally expressive ways. In fact, the Anlo-Ewe people recognize numerous kinds of walking, each of which expresses moral and social qualities; 'a person's character was revealed in his or her walk or mode of comportment: the moral fiber of a person was embodied and expressed in the way that he or she moved' (Geurts 2002, p. 51). These modes of movement and ways of carrying/ expressing oneself are not merely symbolic but, instead, are considered essential qualities of what it means to be a properly socialized Anlo-Ewe person.

Geurts also found that an underlying concept of *nlo*, curling up or turning oneself inward, is a kind of emplacement that is both culturally and psychologically significant for Anlo-Ewe people:

> Nlo becomes 'real' in a time and space between body, mind, self, other, subject, and object (rather than exclusively in one of those domains). Such indeterminacy as is illustrated here is an essential aspect of one's existence in the 'lived world of perceptual phenomena' that constitutes Anlo ethnoscapes and Anlo selves.
>
> (Geurts 2000, p. 120)

This bodily movement and spatial experience is a 'mostly unconscious dimension of self-processes in Anlo contexts' (p. 120). The idea and experience of *nlo* distills the tensions between dualisms such as freedom and exhaustion, joy and sorrow, and humor and grief, although Geurts notes that the Anlo-Ewe people tend toward the more melancholic (pp. 120–121). *Nlo* is a kind of rounded-ness (literally) that brings about a centeredness in the domains of emotion, intuition, imagination, perception, and sensation and includes a sense of the migratory and struggling past of their ancestors. Other thematized cultural motifs are also central to self-processes and, if someone doesn't attend to these motifs, he or she fails to develop a sense of identity grounded in these cultural themes (p. 145).

Of course, all cultures have motifs and themes that its people are expected to internalize in order to be counted as enculturated. But my point is that the concepts of seselelame and *nlo* are two features of Anlo-Ewe culture that suggests that these people conceptualize self, embodiment, and identity differently than do Westerners. Consider that a central way in which the production of Anlo-Ewe identity occurs is through ritual, something largely lost in twenty-first century post-industrialist Western societies. Ritual presents an embodied pathway for persons to internalize social identity and ancestor relations. Geurts explains that ritual allows persons emotionally to encounter ancestors, thus incorporating the past into their identity and affirming a continuity of past and present cultural norms. To summarize, in studying the culture of Anlo-Ewe people, Geurts found that 'well-being is not achieved within the confines of the individual … Selves, in fact, in West African contexts are very "porous"' by which Geurts means that the self is open to influences and 'exists only in the sense that she is related to other (animal, human, and divine) beings' (Geurts 2002, pp. 169–170). 'All the components of persons, or the "parts inside of persons," are to a certain extent the province of ancestral spirits' (Geurts 2002, p. 176). Anlo-Ewe culture, thus, stands as an example of the culturally constructed aspects of identity that may challenge prevailing Western conceptions as reviewed above. It highlights the problem for psychiatry that what counts as identity disturbance in one culture may be quite normal and acceptable in another.

Studies show that the identity construct differs from culture to culture (Markus *et al.* 1997). 'Particularized senses of the self – self-concepts and individuated identities – are always grounded in the complex of consensual understandings and customary behavioral routines relevant to being a self in a given sociocultural and historical context' (Markus *et al.* 1997, p. 15). In European American contexts, evidence of malleability and variability in one's identity is discouraged and even challenged (p. 24). In contrast, research shows that, in Japanese culture, the relationship, not the individual, is the functional unit of the psyche and that the content of identity for Japanese people is contingent upon those relationships. Identity disturbance, it would follow, is also culturally inflected.

1.7 Conclusion: The pain of identity troubles

I now distill the problems with the construct within psychiatry that have emerged from the discussion.

First, identity difficulties are unlikely universally to be experienced as feelings of emptiness and uncertainty about values and commitments. The notion of the self as unified and stable is a product of a particular era with its own background, ontological commitments, and ethos. Drawing upon the language of John Sadler, I suggest that the prevailing identity construct used to distinguish healthy identity from unhealthy is embedded in ontological value entailments (Sadler 2005, p. 217). If the boundary between healthy and troubled identities is determined in part by ontological values that vary from culture to culture, it is difficult to see the appropriateness or usefulness of a scientific criterion for identity disturbance. How can the criterion be tested? Standardized?

Secondly, Wilkinson-Ryan and Westen's findings suggest that 'painful incoherence' is the most salient factor for BPD patients who show symptoms of identity disturbance. But now we can press the question, Why is 'incoherence' painful? Is it inherently painful? Or are identity troubles a response to conflicts with society? I have argued that some aspects of the BPD diagnosis are based on assumptions that are Western constructs. Marie Crowe argues that the feelings of identity struggles and distress found in patients diagnosed with BPD are more accurately thought of as expressions of shame; what is now called 'identity disturbance' shows up, in her interviews with patients, as a discrepancy between the patient's ideal self and how she thinks she is being perceived by others. One patient says, 'I just want people to accept me and to like me … I set very high standards for myself … I've got to do the right thing all the time. I want people to see me as someone who can do OK' (Crowe 2004, p. 331). Attempts to satisfy others shape patients' behaviors, and failures to satisfy others lead to anger, depression, and intensified shame.[5] In the light of my previous discussion of conflicting and demanding gendered expectations for women, it may be difficult to determine when feelings of identity distress are grounded in social norms and ensuing conflicts and when something pathological is occurring. As Sadler argues, clinicians face significant difficulties when trying to distinguish between a person's response to adverse social conditions from her response to an 'internal dysfunction' (Sadler 2005, pp. 208–209). Making such

---

[5] While I think Crowe's suggestion is interesting that the symptoms of BPD are better explained by shame than by a personality disorder, I do not take up this line of argument because my primary aim in this book is not to provide an alternative diagnosis for patients but to probe assumptions and problems in the current diagnosis and its corresponding treatment approaches.

a determination is burdensome and impractical, given how hopelessly muddled is the question of the 'location' of distress (p. 209).

The third point is related to the second one but concerns how to frame distress that is severe enough to interfere with a person's daily life. In section 1.6, I suggested that materialism and the socialization of females are two factors that contribute to feelings of emptiness and uncertainty about values, meaning making, and relationships. These factors suggest that at least some causes of distress are social. Yet feelings of emptiness and uncertainty about one's values, aims, and commitments have been 'medicalized,' which is to take a concept and constrain it with medical rather than social meanings (Sadler 2005, p. 238). The problem with medicalizing distress and suffering is that it blames victims of suffering for the problems of society (Sadler 2005, p. 238). Sadler urges that distress and suffering be contextualized within the social and cultural circumstances that create stress on devalued groups such as women of all colors.

For these reasons, I conclude that an understanding of the self as a cultural construct is crucially important in working with BPD patients. Problems and questions of how to understand identity disturbance must be contextualized to cultures, norms of gender, and the effects of materialism and technologies on the construct of identity. The issue should be: what does it mean for this person, in this culture, (a) to have an identity that (b) is disturbed? What piece of the identity is disturbed independent of the intersections of identity and culture? Addressing these philosophical/clinical questions will undoubtedly make treatment more difficult – but if it is better to think more complexly about a feature of BPD, then 'think more complexly' is the clinician's task. Nevertheless, therapists can validate a patient's feeling of emptiness by contextualizing it as a cultural phenomenon. Situating emptiness this way helps to normalize feelings of emptiness while at the same time working on managing distress and pain that stem from those feelings. I take up this issue in Chapter 9 when discussing empathy.

Chapter 2

The problem with too much anger

2.1 Vignette

> A concerned mother called me to raise the issue of whether some further, perhaps
> different, treatment might be needed for her daughter. I responded by saying that
> I would talk with the patient about this concern and would get back to her. After
> talking with her daughter, I suggested that she call her mother while she was still there
> and could participate on another line. The patient promptly began a lengthy diatribe
> at her mother for interfering and poor judgment … After trying unsuccessfully to
> interject some comments, I put my finger across my lips and went, "Shh," to my
> patient. She ragefully slammed down the telephone and left.

> (Gunderson 1984, pp.110–111)

How are we to view this patient's anger? Over-the-top? Inappropriate? Did the
psychiatrist provoke her anger? Was the anger warranted?

This patient is diagnosed with borderline personality disorder (BPD). Patients
with BPD are considered difficult to interact with in part because of their anger
(Gunderson 2001; Linehan 1993). Inappropriate or intense anger is one of the
criteria for BPD: 'frequent displays of temper, constant anger, recurrent physical fights' (DSM-IV-TR 2000, p. 710). If we are correctly to identify when this
criterion is present, we need to know the difference between pathological and
reasonable anger and what norms govern the distinction. I will argue four
things (1) that anger is a form of communication that requires acknowledgement from the listener; (2) that BPD anger is dispositional (and often dispositionally dysfunctional), but that a patient also can have occurrent anger that is
reasonable; (3) that failing to acknowledge BPD anger risks worsening their
problems; and (4) that assessments of BPD anger draw upon contextual norms
for expression of emotion that may impede clinicians giving appropriate
acknowledgement. I begin with a philosophical discussion of anger.

2.2 What is anger?

Anger is a moral emotion, which is to say that moral judgments are normatively
paired with particular emotional responses (D'Arms and Jacobson 1994, p. 748).

Marcia Linehan describes emotions as 'full systems responses. That is, they are integrated patterns of experiential, cognitive, and expressive, as well as physiological, responses' (Linehan 1993, p. 68). Grammatically, a person is 'angry at' someone or 'about' something. As Larry May argues, anger is stimulated by a sense of injury; the object of anger repels (May 1998, pp. 18–19). May suggests that anger is a kind of reactive assessment, and it may be rudimentary, as when one thinks that it has taken another too long to respond to a question but still involves some kind of conscious assessment (May 1998, p. 19).

To elaborate on the concept of anger, I draw upon the work by Frye and Austin on language, as well as previous research of my own (Potter 2000). 'Being angry at someone,' Frye writes, 'is somewhat like a speech act in that it has a certain conventional force whereby it sets people up in a certain sort of orientation to each other; and like a speech act, it cannot "come off" if it does not get uptake' (Frye 1983). In Part II of this book, I introduce the concept of uptake as a virtue and explain how it is useful to clinicians to think of giving uptake as a virtue. Here, I analyze the concept as it relates to anger.

Austin (1975) introduced the concept of uptake to characterize the engagement of the listener in order to secure the meaning of a speech act: when the listener accepts another's speech act and gives it the conventional understanding, the listener has given the speaker uptake. For example, my promise to you can only be said to be successful when you understand my speech act as one in which I place myself under obligation to you (Austin 1975, p. 571). Your recognition of my speech act as a promise is the uptake.

Uptake, then, occurs when the listening party reorients herself to the communicator and the relation between the two of them 'comes off' with an appropriate response. As I discuss elsewhere (Potter 2002, 2000), oftentimes expressions of anger are acts of claiming that call for a response to a person's claim that she has been wronged; giving uptake to anger requires that the audience acknowledges (1) that a claim is being made, and (2) that the claim is asserting the speaker's worth.

> To get angry is to claim implicitly that one is a certain sort of being, a being which can ... stand in a certain relation and position a propos the being one is angry at. One claims that one is in certain ways and dimensions respectable. One makes claims upon respect.
>
> (Frye 1983)

The point is that anger is relational; it has a logic that involves perceived wrongdoer and wronged. As such, a respectful way to respond to anger would be to give it uptake even if it turns out that the angry person's perception of a wrong was incorrect. Anger is not always 'about' injury, of course; it could be caused by physiological responses to frustration or stress. I am talking about a particular kind of anger.

May's and Frye's work is useful in thinking about BPD anger in three ways. First, May suggests that it should be approached as a reactive assessment, which idea emphasizes the cognitive aspect of getting angry. Although anger can be triggered by unconscious associations, it also involves perception, belief, and interpretation and cannot be reduced to the unconscious.

Second, an application of their work to BPD patients suggests that some of those patients may be trying to make a claim about a moral right that they think has been violated. Patients are often characterized as having an exaggerated sense of entitlement. When viewed this way, their attempts to assert moral rights are viewed as irrational. An ethical response to expressions of anger includes an attempt to understand what sort of moral claim the patient is making and not to assume that the patient is exaggerating her entitlements. In fact, giving uptake properly is a virtue of its own and is bound up with trustworthiness (cf. Potter 2002); hence, appropriate responses to patient anger are part of clinician trustworthiness.

Third, at the heart of expressed anger is an attempt to assert one's respect. An alternative way of thinking about borderline anger is that the patient is asserting her worth as a self-respecting human being in the face of perceived injury or insult. As Jeffrie Murphy says, '… If I count morally as much as anyone else (as surely I do), a failure to resent moral injuries done to me is a failure to care about the moral value incarnate in my own moral personality' (Murphy 1982, p. 505).When a patient's anger is not given uptake, the patient is treated as if she has not communicated; the listener, by refusing even to consider the patient's attempt to orient their relationship as injurer and injured, demeans the patient's assertion of self-worth. In sum, I am suggesting that the patient's anger should be given uptake because to do so is to recognize her moral worth as a person who is attempting to uphold her own value in the face of perceived hurt.

Of course, patients diagnosed with BPD and the rest of us can get it wrong about anger in a variety of ways, and it is to this point that I now turn.

2.3 Anger, extremes, and dispositional anger

From an Aristotelian framework, our aim should be to develop a disposition such that we neither overdo nor underdo our responses (Aristotle 1999). Anger can be inappropriate not only if it lasts too long, or is too vehement for the situation, but also if the target of one's anger is not the person who did the wrongdoing. On the other hand, Aristotle (like Murphy) believes that not having enough anger is also blameworthy. 'For such a person seems to be insensible and to feel no pain, and since he is not angered, he does not seem to be the sort to defend himself. Such willingness to accept insults to oneself and to overlook insults to one's family and friends is slavish' (Aristotle 1999, 1126a5–1126a10). Aristotle names the mean the virtue of 'mildness,' which is 'being undisturbed, not led by feeling, but irritated wherever reason prescribes, and for the length of time it prescribes' (Aristotle 1999, 1125b35).

The judgment of an 'excess' is located in terms of appropriate responses relative to the context, where the mean for anger is the intermediate condition between excess and deficiency in a particular situation. One reason why it's so difficult to get clear on what counts as excessive anger in BPD patients is that the DSM models are decontextualized. But judgments of extreme or inappropriate anger cannot be made from an abstract point of view. Diagnostic manuals may treat criteria such as inappropriate anger as simple facts, when they actually require evaluative judgments. Furthermore, extreme or inappropriate anger is not necessarily pathological; it may be just a mistake.

On a standard analysis, anger can be either occurrent or dispositional. An occasional expression of excessive, deficient, or inappropriate anger is not so much a cause of concern; the important question is what we have a tendency to do when faced with perceived insults and injuries. If we have a tendency to vent our anger at safe targets rather than the object of our anger, or to explain away all insults as benign and unimportant, we have a disposition toward anger that is flawed.

Excessive or inappropriate anger does not seem to be the only problematic emotion for many BPD patients. But as Linehan says, 'they often have difficulty regulating the entire pattern of responses associated with particular emotional states' (1993, p. 68). All their negative emotions appear to be dispositional, too. But because of the tendency to associate current injuries with past wounds, BPD anger appears to be only dispositionally maladaptive where, in fact, three issues exist: dispositional anger that is hard-wired, a disposition to bring past anger into the present, and occurrent anger in the present. Here the standard picture of dispositional or occurrent anger is too simple – both because it is most often a doubling of the present with the past and because norms underlying assessments of anger are themselves complex.

I have indicated that expressions of anger require uptake – but a number of things prevent clinicians from doing so. The next sections review some of those obstacles and indicate what is involved in giving uptake to someone whose disposition regarding anger is maladaptive.

2.4 The doubling effect of injury on anger

One difficulty in giving uptake to BPD anger is that it often isn't clear what the anger is 'about.' Many clinicians posit BPD anger as a regression to primitive defenses such as 'denial, acting out, and projection which prevent the patient's recognition of the feeling response and its reason' (Gunderson 2001, p. 53; Gunderson 1984, p. 35; Kernberg 1984) and, by definition, primitive defenses are irrational. If a clinician assumes that a patient's anger is coming from past wounds, the patient may seem unreasonable when she insists she is angry with the clinician for hurt the clinician inflicted. Of course, many clinicians distinguish between the actual relationship between clinician and patient, and the transference relationship that the real relationship makes possible. But others are not so insightful and sensitive to this distinction, as the literature suggests, so it is important to bring these philosophical points to light.

The problem with interpreting all BPD anger as regressive is that it denies the possibility that a person has both warranted, real-time anger and maladaptive anger in response to the past. Linehan encourages clinicians to see the patient's anger as reasonable, although perhaps mixed with other emotions. She distinguishes 'primary' (authentic) emotions from 'secondary' (learned) ones. Secondary emotions are 'reactions to primary cognitive appraisals and emotional responses; they are the end products of chains of feelings and thoughts.' Maladaptive responses become interwoven with valid ones (Linehan 1993, p. 227).

This is what I am calling the doubling effect of injury on anger. Although a patient may have maladaptive anger dispositionally, she may still be able to have occurrent anger that is warranted. Real-time occurrent anger can be an echo of past wounds. Developmental theories of BPD suggest that patients carry deep early childhood wounds that are associated with their dysfunctional and disruptive behaviors. In fact, Linehan argues that 'the amelioration of unendurable emotional pain is always suspected as one of the primary motivational factors in borderline dysfunctional behavior' (Linehan 1993, p. 265; see also p. 59). The woundedness underlying anger must be given uptake in order for patients to heal. As Linehan points out, it may be difficult to uncover old wounds partly because the patient herself is confused about her feelings. My concern here, though, is that in viewing real-time anger as merely symbolic of past wounds, clinicians may miss important communicative moments. When clinicians focus exclusively on the irrationality or distorted views of the patient, therapy is undermined (Linehan 1993, p. 229). And, in fact, inattention to real-time anger may spark a destructive pattern in that it provokes more hostility and anger when a perceived real-time injury is not taken seriously. The difficulty for these patients is that real-time anger is amplified by past wounds, and the intensity may make it difficult for the patient to regulate it. But amplification from doubling doesn't mean that it is not important to respond to real-time occurrent anger independently. Precisely because it is a doubled effect and not only an old wound, both injuries need to be addressed. Clinicians can assist patients in distinguishing these types of anger, thus helping them to gain insight into the various sources of their anger.

In the next sections, I focus on that part of BPD anger that is an assessment in real time.

2.5 **What impedes giving uptake to real-time anger?**

The kind of anger we are considering is a cognitively mediated response to perceived injury or injustice. I have argued that some of those injuries or insults occur in the present moment and that BPD anger cannot all be reduced to pathological responses to past events. So how do we distinguish between anger that hits the mean, extremes of anger, and pathological anger? May suggests that anger that hits the mean would be '*in some sense reasonable*' (May 1998, 12; emphasis added). That is, from the perspective of the subject, anger is a reasonable response to a perceived violation *of a norm that the subject accepts* (May 1998, 15; emphasis added).

I will note three things that interfere with giving uptake when considering the idea of 'reasonableness.'

One is that I may be angry and believe the anger is reasonable and appropriate but others do not. People differ considerably in what they count as a violation or an injustice. Norms for behavior are not necessarily shared. Furthermore, perspective affects how a moral wrong is viewed or even whether or not it is acknowledged. For example, many people would defend telling a lie who would nevertheless object to being told one (Bok 1978). Finally, the social and cultural groupings of power are in a stronger position to determine and enforce social norms, such that the norms of the powerful dominate our assessments and others' behavior. According to Dyke and Dyke, the privileged center – defined by those at the intersection of the privileged with respect to nationality, class, race, gender, and sexuality – accrue advantages of psychological, motivational, educational, and social networks and produce and reproduce 'a complex of shared values, assumptions, standards, and practices to which all others become entrained' (2002, pp. 79–80). This complex forms the dominant culture and its norms. Dominant norms influence what can be expressed and how and by whom. In Chapter 1, we examined norms of identity; in this chapter, we are considering norms regarding anger.

Anger, I have suggested, is an assessment that one's moral rights have been violated. One form that takes is in terms of norms of relationship, where expectations about those norms have been thwarted. Let us contemplate, for a moment, what norms of interaction might be operational for a patient that would make her anger seem reasonable to her if a norm is violated. Possible norms:

Norm: People ought not to appear bored or restless when I am talking.
Norm: People ought to listen attentively when I am talking.

Norm: People ought not to slough me off on others when I am appealing to them for help.

Norm: People should be careful not to automatically discount or suspect me when I explain things to them or express needs.

Norm: People should take me seriously when I say I am frantic and desperate.

Norm: People ought to go out of their way to reassure me that they are not abandoning me if they are planning a holiday.

What is the status of these norms? With the exception of the last one, I suspect many people (in relatively good mental health) subscribe to them. Of course, these norms are applied in different contexts with different results; I too expect to be listened to when I talk to my close friend, but I don't feel particularly insulted when my students are bored. Still, that such norms are reasonable, from the point of view of the patient, is an important clue to assessment and response of borderline anger. 'All norms ... are norms of warrant—they're about what it makes sense to think, to want, or to feel' (D'Arms and Jacobson 1994, p. 742). I acknowledge that BPD patients can expect too much and that some BPD anger leads to loss of control and so is unreasonable. It is important, though, not to confuse impassioned anger with out-of-control rage. Anger is a passion, and fear of passions may prompt us to judge them as dangerous when they are merely expressions of strong feeling (Fisher 2002).

My point is that a failure to give uptake to the patient's sense that a norm or moral right has been violated is to dismiss her norms and expectations as invalid. Such a move cannot be made *a priori* to giving uptake; we cannot judge whether a real-time injury actually occurred until we have explored that possibility. And genuine engagement in exploring possible real-time injuries requires us to be willing to subject our own norms to scrutiny and to take into consideration that the patient's norms may be, in some sense, reasonable or understandable .

Secondly, norms alone don't tell us whether or not an emotion is appropriate for the context. Some situations may call for extreme expressions of emotion even when the governing social norms encourage moderation. The anger of BPD patients is often described as an overly sensitive response to slights and inattention, or a reaction to approaching loss or abandonment. If we disregard the experience of double-woundedness – that what the patient is reacting to in the present is an echo of a wound in the past – then perhaps we might view her as overly sensitive. But that way of thinking about patients' sensitivity risks being dismissive of her situatedness in the context of her current therapeutic relationship.

A psychoanalytic way of framing the complicated interaction between patient and therapist when it concerns BPD patient anger is in terms of projective identification. Projection is a primitive defense mechanism by which a person externalizes negative feelings about oneself through ascribing them to another (Adler 1985.) Projective identification occurs when the person doing the projecting induces the other to take on those projections – meaning that the other person behaves in ways the projector unconsciously expects or fears (Cashdan 1988; cf. also Kernberg 1967). For example, Sally projects onto her partner the negative representations she holds of her mother, and her partner starts to fulfill those negative projections by becoming 'bad' in ways that map onto Sally's beliefs and feelings about her mother. Sheldon Cashdan explains that the difference between projection and projective identification is that the former is a mental act that may not involve any response from the other about the projection whereas projective identification is a dynamic within a relationship (Cashdan 1988). Projection and projective identification, along with splitting (discussed in Chapter 1) are three core primitive defense mechanisms that work together to help people cope with negative feelings about themselves and others by externalizing negativity. They are considered primitive because, although they are developmentally useful, they impede mature psychological health. I bring up the process of projective identification because it is a phenomenon found in therapeutic relationships when the patient has insufficiently dealt with unconscious and internalized negative experiences. In particular, projective identification may occur when a BPD patient is angry about matters unrelated to therapy but directs her anger toward her therapist. The therapist might, understandably, feel unfairly attacked and unjustifiably blamed. If the therapist becomes defensive or even subtly rejecting of the patient's anger, the therapist may exhibit the negative or bad behavior that the patient has projected onto the therapist. Such projective identification is counterproductive to the therapeutic process because the patient does not then need to address her own conflicted or ambivalent feelings and beliefs. Skillful handling of the patient's anger thus requires appropriate uptake which, in turn, requires that the therapist contextualize the anger and the therapist's response within not only the therapeutic relationship but also to the patient's present and past outside of therapy.

However we theoretically frame the messiness of BPD anger within the therapeutic relationship, we would do well to draw some philosophical distinctions when making judgments about the status of a patient's anger. I follow a distinction drawn by D'Arms and Jacobson: even if a feeling is undesirable (based on norms), this is not grounds for calling it unwarranted (D'Arms and Jacobson 1994, p. 744). Belief is an integral part of emotion. When we feel anger toward someone or about something, it is because we hold a belief about the person or action or situation, and we represent it to ourselves in a way that gives rise to anger. Warrant is determined by the content of the belief component of the emotion; an emotion is unwarranted when its belief component is unjustified' (D'Arms and Jacobson 1994, p. 748). Still, one person's warrant may be another person's 'unwarrant'; warrant must be understood from the patient's point of view but the fact that the patient believes she is warranted in a belief does not make it justified by itself. Warrant is a social accomplishment.

The point is that one's anger or rage may be extreme and therefore outside the norms for anger but that leaves open the question of whether the anger is warranted. The clinician must also establish what beliefs the patient and clinician each are holding and consider to what extent those beliefs are warranted. A problem in giving uptake occurs when the clinician assumes the dysfunctionality of her BPD patient and so has difficulty seeing the patient as a sometimes-reasonable moral agent. Talking about the beliefs that underlie anger is one way to give uptake to the anger without exacerbating it and may allow the patient to explore other feelings. It may also allow the clinician to identify beliefs and attitudes that are inadvertently contributing to a patient's echo experience of injury.

But a further difficulty arises when framing appropriate anger in terms of reasonableness – because that norm is based on a theory of rationality that is biased. Reasonableness is assessed similarly to the 'reasonable man' standard used in law (cf. Prosser 1971). But this ideal itself is gendered, as legal scholars argue (cf. Hubin and Haely 1999; Raigrodski 1999). The reasonable man is an idealized abstraction and is alleged to be generic but, as so often happens, the generic person turns out to be male.

The problem is not new: since the time of the Pythagoreans, rationality has been linked with maleness and emotionality with femaleness (cf. Whitbeck 1973). Moreover, the idea that women are not in control of their emotions is not unique to BPD or other mentally disordered women. If appropriate anger is anger that is reasonable, and women by nature are believed to be irrational, then it follows that women's anger will not be perceived as reasonable. And BPD patients are 75% female (DSM IV-TR 2000.) This is the third problem in evaluating anger as reasonable, inappropriate, or extreme.

2.6 **Anger and gender norms**

Rom Harré argues that understanding emotions requires that we attend to local systems of rights and obligations, and value in particular contexts (Harré 1986, p. 6). 'Instead of asking the question, "What is anger?"' Harré writes, 'we would do well to begin by asking, "How is the word 'anger,' and other expressions that cluster around it, actually used in this or that cultural milieu and type of episode?"' (1986, pp. 4–5). While I will still ask the standard philosophical question of what anger is, I think Harré is right.

I pursue these ideas by examining norms for behavior as they concern expressions of anger by women.

As May points out, '[a]nger and rage are so commonly expressed by young adult males that we all come to expect it' (May 1998, p. 8). Not so with women. Frye argues that women's anger at moral injustices done to them do not get taken seriously and respectfully; instead, women's anger gets trivialized, pathologized, mocked, and ignored. 'Deprived of uptake, the woman's anger is left as just a burst of expression of individual feeling. As a social act, an act of communication, it just doesn't happen' (Frye 1983, p. 89).

Our conventions of language have different norms for giving uptake to women than to men. In particular, the norms for uptake are gendered regarding expressions of anger. Women are not supposed to get angry, or women get provoked by trivial events, and so on. When it comes to women's claims of injustices and injuries, women are told to stop 'playing the victim,' to stop blaming others for their plight, and to take responsibility for their lives (cf. Lamb 1996). In fact, according to Linehan, 'The problem for many borderline patients is not the overexperience and expression of anger, but rather the underexpression of it; that is, they are anger-phobic' (Linehan 1993, p. 356). What they fear is rejection due to their expression of strong emotion. In fact, fear of strong emotions, especially anger, is a more general problem for women. It is a recognized social phenomenon that girls and women are not taught that it is sometimes appropriate to be angry or what appropriate expressions of it look like (cf. van Daalen-Smith 2008; Cox *et al.* 1999; Brown and Gilligan 1992). Some are unable even to identify what anger feels like.

As I have suggested, cultural analyses reveal that we accord praise and blame for expressions of anger differentially depending on gender. Linehan reflects that whether a BPD patient's behavior is interpreted as angry depends on who is doing the interpreting (1993, p. 70). 'The overinterpretation of anger and hostile intent, however, can itself generate hostility and anger' (Linehan 1993, p. 71).

Claims about gender norms for anger and other problems do not eliminate the need for concern about BPD anger. Excessive or inappropriate anger can be dysfunctional because problems with anger can cause other life difficulties (Linehan 1993, p. 71) and can be disturbing or disruptive to the patients themselves. But Linehan, too, recognizes the gender norms at work in assessing anger in BPD patients: with respect to women, 'even minor expressions of anger may be interpreted as aggression. For example, behavior that is labeled as "assertive" in men may be labeled "aggressive" in women. Perceived aggression begets retaliatory aggression, and thus the cycle of interpersonal conflict is born' (Linehan 1993, p. 71).

Women are in a double-bind when it comes to anger. If they are vehement in their expressions of anger, they may be viewed as pathologically angry.

If they are already viewed as 'too angry,' then their denying that they are angry is proof of regression. What the patient takes to be a real-time provocation can be interpreted as evidence of acting out or projection and, given that standards for rationality are themselves gendered, it is often difficult for a female patient to make her case that a present hurt or injustice was, indeed, done to her. Clinicians run the risk of assuming that excessive anger is so much a part of a patient's character that she is unable ever to be reasonably angry. A patient's sense of herself as an adequate reasoner and moral agent is at stake here, and it is important to give her real-time anger uptake.

Let me return to the opening vignette now and tell you what really happened-because the clinician did give uptake to the patient's anger, and the outcome was constructive.

Vignette

A concerned mother called me to raise the issue of whether some further, perhaps different, treatment might be needed for her daughter. I responded by saying that I would talk with the patient about this concern and would get back to her. After talking with her daughter, I suggested that she call her mother while she was still there and could participate on another line. The patient promptly began a lengthy diatribe at her mother for interfering and poor judgment. **It was late and I was tired**. After trying unsuccessfully to interject some comments, I put my finger across my lips and went, "Shh," to my patient. She ragefully slammed down the telephone and left. She subsequently told me how she felt demeaned, how she felt I was taking her mother's side, and that she considered not coming back. **I acknowledged that it had been an unfortunate indication of my impatience and a better means of getting to the issues I felt needed to be addressed should have been used**.

(Gunderson 1984, pp. 110–111; emphasis added)

The clinician acknowledged a real-time provocation and injury to which the patient was responding with anger. After admitting his role in the troubled interaction, he reported that the session went on to explore other times the patient felt demeaned. This simple acknowledgement emphasizes the primacy of taking real-time BPD anger seriously and respectfully, even when its expression may in part hark back to other wrongs, and even when the size of it may seem out of place. Taking responsibility for even minor current provocations can advance therapy and build a stronger therapeutic alliance.

2.7 Conclusion

Anger has a present as well as a past. To understand it and assess its appropriateness, clinicians need to contextualize patients' anger in relation not only to the patient's past injuries but in relation to possible present ones. I have argued that clinicians need to give uptake to the anger of BPD patients and to consider it as possibly warranted in real-time as well as doubled. Giving uptake should include considering the beliefs and injury behind the anger. Clinicians will do best to acknowledge occasions when their attitudes and assumptions may, in fact, be slighting or injuring their BPD patients. Giving uptake to real-time anger as *prima facie* distinct from past wounds defuses it and opens up a space to talk about past wounds, and ways in which a present time injury is an echo of the patient's past.

Anger has a present and a past, but it also has a future because anger implies hope (Sharpe 2003, p. 35).[1] Anger says, 'I still believe in myself; I am self-respecting; I believe in a future in which the injuries I sustain are not all-encompassing, and the hope I bear is that my anger gets taken seriously by you.'

---

[1] 'Chris felt sick with fear and anger; no, not anger—anger implied hope; hatred'.

Chapter 3

Rocky relationships

3.1 **An example**

Anthony Walker, an intern who had just gotten married, describes a conversation with his new wife [diagnosed with BPD] when he announced he was going for a run:

> "I am off, darling," I told Jacqueline, who lay burrowed in her duvet.
> "Where to?" she asked.
> "For a run. Look at this, I am getting fat." I wobbled my gut in front of her, laughing.
> "So what?"
> "What do you mean?"
> "So what if you're getting fat?"
> "I need to lose some weight."
> "Who are you trying to impress?"
> "Nobody, it's just a healthy thing to do. Anyway, my pants are getting tight."
> "What's wrong with all you men? You think that you have to have rock hard bodies to get the chicks. That's not what women want. That's not what I want. I want you to take care of me. I want you to make so much money that I never have to work, and that we can go to restaurants whenever we want. I don't want some pansy prancing around in his tights."
> "What's gotten into you? This isn't some vanity trip. I'm just going for a run."
> "So it is more important to you to go for a run than to be with me?"
> "What are you talking about? I am with you. I'll be back in half an hour."
> Jacqueline took a half-empty wineglass from the nightstand and smashed it to the ground. "What the hell are you doing to me? You promised me that you would never leave." I shuddered and stepped back from her. She started to cry. "You are doing that now. You promised that you would never leave me." I went to hold her.

(Walker 2001, pp. 54–55)

Walker's anecdote about the escalation to desperation and volatility his wife expresses when she interprets his plan to go for a run as abandonment is a common one in relationships where one partner has borderline tendencies. His story relates the agony and confusion that sometimes comes from being in a romantic or coupling relationship with a BPD patient. Given the problems associated with BPD, it is not surprising that these patients often have troubled and tumultuous relationships. The doubling effect of anger, for example, can take a toll on relationships; feelings of emptiness can make connection with others difficult. This chapter examines the difficulty with interpersonal relationships that are a common experience of many BPD patients while situating such difficulties in a larger social context.

Being co-participants in interpersonal relationships is a central part of living a flourishing life (Reis and Gable 2003). As Aristotle (1999) says, 'no one would choose to live without friends even if he had all the other goods.' The assumption is that we all live better lives when we share our lives with others and that a life without close friends or intimates is an impoverished one. It is a reasonable assumption. But for some BPD patients, the problem is not that they are loners or recluses or introverts. Instead, the problem is said to be that their relationships tend to extremes. Some BPD patients form intense relationships and then sever those relationships suddenly and violently. They seem not to be able to find a middle ground between passionate valorization of the other and hurtful detachment. So, on the one hand, first-person accounts of relationship troubles, such as Walker narrates (2001; cf. Reiland (2004)), highlight the distress BPD patients experience – and the distress that they inflict on their loved ones. On the other hand, as I argue, cultural norms and gendered expectations of relationships shape both the ways in which women experience and practice relationality and, when women deviate from those norms, how their behavior is evaluated.

Criterion 2 for BPD is 'a pattern of unstable and intense interpersonal relationships characterized by alternating between extremes of idealization and devaluation' (DSM 2000, p. 710). In this chapter, I primarily focus on the values and assumptions that undergird that criterion, that is, on the value of relationship, the norms that govern relationship, and the quality of connection needed to sustain flourishing relationships. In the next section (3.2), I discuss some of the main characteristics in relationships, namely, intimacy, trust, connection, and repair. My choice in discussing those characteristics shouldn't be taken as claims about necessary and sufficient conditions for quality relationships; instead, I selected aspects of relationships that I think may give special trouble to BPD women. Surely, I am missing others, but this provides a conceptual starting point. In section 3.3, I compare belongingness with a desire for 'home' and what is, in clinical circles, called desperate love. I draw on metaphors of home and homesickness and bring in Plato's myth from the *Symposium* that we humans are always searching for our 'other half.' Section 3.4 provides findings about the different expectations for women in a relationship than for men and explains how the last several decades have led to an embracing of a female ethic, called the ethic of care, that emphasizes relationality (the idea that we are first and foremost selves in relation to others and secondarily are autonomous individuals – a descriptive claim with heavy normative dimensions), being in relationship, and maintaining personal attachments. Section 3.4 presents a critique of such a view. I argue that first, it burdens women with the work of 'repair' in relationships (Spelman 2004); second, it valorizes attachment at the expense of protecting women from traumatic relationships; and third, it sets up a negative evaluation of women who are not good at something taken to be 'natural' to women's relationships.

3.2 Intimacy, connection, and repair

In this section, I consider some of the central aspects of being in relationship, with the aim of normalizing, to some extent, the quality of relationship which is thought to be typical of BPD patients. In thinking about these qualities, though, I do not want to diminish the very real strain that people face, as in the opening case of Walker and his wife. Jacqueline's fear of being abandoned does seem to be extreme, given how reassuring Walker seems to be. Still, I think it is worthwhile to examine more closely some of the norms of relationship. The aim, I remind readers, is to see what norms may shape expectations of BPD women and also what norms may shape evaluations of them in the clinical setting.

3.2.1 Intimacy and connection

Vaughn Sinclair and Sharon Dowdy (2005), citing earlier work by Weiss, identify six aspects of social relationships that are important for well-being: a sense of belonging; a provision for intimacy; an opportunity to be nurturing; the availability of advice and guidance; a reassurance of worth and accomplishments; and a reliable and consistent person in one's life (Sinclair and Dowdy 2005, p. 194). Emotional intimacy is but one kind of intimacy (others include sexual intimacy, affectional intimacy, and intellectual intimacy), yet it, along with affectional intimacy, is perhaps foundational to well-being.

There are many characteristics that need to be considered in intimate relations. We have needs, expectations, and hopes that center on the intimate one, yet we may feel ambivalent. We long for companionship, affirmation of our centrality to the intimate, yet we also require boundaries and space. We want to be empathetic and empathized with, yet we may also find ourselves judging the intimate one and being criticized by him or her. We ache for harmony and a sense of unity, and we must also deal with difference and conflict.

I relate the idea of intimacy to the concept of connection. A normative notion of intimacy concerns the quality of connection we experience. Being close to another, whether an intimate other or a clinician, is an ongoing process of sustaining connection and repairing relational damage. I define connection as being with another person in whatever feelings and thoughts that person is having, seeing that person in the moment, and allowing the other to be with you in that way as well (Potter 2002). Staying connected requires being able to keep trusting the other, even through difficulties (within reason, as I discuss below).

Knowledge of other people – and the closeness that comes along with it – includes cognitive, emotional, and behavioral closeness and is structured by a complex web of expectations, hopes, memories, caring, and trust (Martin 1993, p. 501). One way that we convey information about ourselves and receive it from others is through 'intimate talk.' While I do not put too much weight on disclosure (we communicate through tactile means, showing emotions, and just being together), it is important to appreciate that revealing ourselves to another (however we do that, and whether it is deliberate or not) makes us feel vulnerable, and so, in order to be willing to take the risks involved in being more vulnerable or vulnerable in ways we haven't been before, we need to have signs of the other's trustworthiness (Strikwerda and May 1992, pp. 101 and 103). Expanding on Reidel's point, I suggest that what marks off the intimate from the less intimate is the quality of connection that exists. Connection, then, turns out to be central to intimacy.

3.2.2 **Trust**

Mutual flourishing is constituted in part by sustained connected close relations. Staying connected in relation requires being able to keep trusting each other. And it requires that the participants be trustworthy in ways particular to the relationship. In other words, if we want to experience sustained connection with particular others, we have to trust and be trusted. I draw on my previous research on trust and trustworthiness (Potter 2002) to expand this discussion. Trust is necessarily given to caregivers when the infant begins life and continues until betrayed or damaged. But infants and children whose trust has been betrayed carry that distrust into future relationships, especially with intimate others. To trust someone is to place something one cares about into the care of another; it involves making oneself vulnerable, especially if what one entrusts is something one cares deeply about (cf. Potter 2002). Trust is distinct from confidence or reliance on another and from contractual relationships in that it leaves open the possibility that the trusted one may not come through in ways the truster hopes.

Intimacy does not require that we be equals, although from the time of Aristotle, many thinkers have recognized the ways in which inequalities can impede intimacy. Govier, for example, excludes parent/adult–child relationships from potential friendships on the grounds that they can never be psychological equals (Govier 1998, p. 27). Govier is right to point to psychological inequalities as another source of inequalities in relationships. Not only must differences in gender, race, or class be navigated in order to sustain intimate relations, but also differences in personal histories. All of us, with our various experiences of hurt and injury in earlier life, bring to relationship histories that complicate our styles of interacting, loving, and giving to one another. Idiosyncrasies and quirks also vary; some people just are reserved, or laid back, or jumpy. (This is not to say that we can't help the way we are, but that there are sometimes physiological factors or long-standing traits that are so deep that they seem 'natural').

Socially shaped positions of inequality, combined with our historical and idiosyncratic selves, make for difficult times within intimate relationships. But they do not make intimacy impossible. Differences in power and equality make it so important to learn how and when to trust, and what is needed to give others as signs of our own trustworthiness.

As Sinclair and Dowdy note, 'emotional intimacy can provide a sense of purpose and belonging' (2005, p. 193). They add that, when people perceive greater emotional intimacy, they are better able to identify what resources are available to them when under stress and that those appraisals, in turn, decrease feelings of powerlessness; people then are less likely to react with high degrees of anxiety and stress to stressful events (Sinclair and Dowdy 2005).

3.2.3 Repair

But, for many people, the fear of being hurt sets up a paradox; the yearning for connection and the fear of being lost in the other can be paralyzing (Jordan 1995, p. 3). Feelings of ambivalence occur occasionally even in the best of relationships, but ambivalence is not an attitude most BPD patients are comfortable with. They are alternately dependent and rejecting, trusting and distrusting.

After clinging to or rejecting the friend, partner, or clinician, the patient may feel the need to repair the damage she has done. Repair is a kind of labor that not only applies to inanimate objects, but also to our bodies, our spirits, and our relationships (Spelman 2004). Healing broken trust and repairing damaged relationships requires that we, first of all, recognize our part in damage done and the need for repair. The BPD patient who recognizes the need for repair has insight but may have a reduced ability to navigate the moral landscape of relationship and personal examination for its fault lines. Repair also involves having personal skills such as self-reflection, personal communication skills, the ability to consider the merits of others' criticism, and the willingness to be honest with ourselves and others. And for the BPD patient to sit comfortably with her flaws (and those of others) takes courage and, probably, a dedicated and trustworthy clinician. (I expand on concepts from this section in Part II of this book).

Jacqueline Walker, the wife in the opening example, exhibits strong distrust of her husband's desire to go on a run. Probably out of insecurity about herself and fear of losing him, she interprets his plan as abandonment. But rather than telling him she's gotten scared and needs reassurance of his ongoing love, she strains their connection by becoming accusatory and needy. She may need to repair the relationship by apologizing for taking her fear to such an extreme that her husband feels unable to fulfill his plan, and he may need to express his resentment while reassuring her that he understands her fears. Whether such gestures are ones that Jacqueline can give and receive may depend on how much her illness is within her control and how successful her treatment has been so far.

3.3 **Belongingness, home, and desperate love**

Like the rest of us, most patients with BPD seek out people with whom they can experience closeness and caring. But many of these women have difficulties in trusting others. The experience of many BPD patients (as well as patients with other diagnoses) is that their trusted caregivers fail them when they are at their most vulnerable – infancy and childhood. Their experience makes it very difficult to trust. Hence, clinicians and intimate others may see testing, insulting, and manipulative behavior as the patient (perhaps unconsciously) determines whether the other person is safe. (But see Chapter 6 for an analysis of manipulativity).

What is interesting is that, once the patient begins to trust, she may throw herself into trusting in ways that are not self-protective, given her now-high expectations. When the entrusted one fails to live up to those high expectations, then that person may become the site of severe accusation as the patient experiences betrayal. As in other forms of dichotomous thinking, the child-like trust/absolute distrust cycle can be trying for all concerned.

As I have argued, intimacy, connection, and mutual trust are central to good relationships. These qualities can provide purpose and belongingness (Sinclair and Dowdy 2005); they are central to our well-being. But having and experiencing a sense of belongingness is difficult for some (perhaps many) people. I discuss the feeling of belongingness by use of metaphors of home and homesickness.

3.3.1 **Belongingness versus home**

One young man describes his time without his girlfriend as 'feeling as if I have no home' (Sperling 1985). He is using the idea of 'home' as a metaphor, and that is how I use it here. 'Home' is a metaphor for a safe place, a place where, as Bernice Johnson Reagon (1983) describes, we are nurtured by others who are like us in relevant ways. It can also be a physical space, where we can 'bar the door' to keep out strangers, dominators, and challengers, and a psychological space for rest and renewal. It is a place, sometimes literally, where we can decide who we are, free of the wider world of conflict, struggle, and defeat. It may also be a psychological place of self-acceptance and rest. Being at home with another person gives us a sense of belongingness and well-being.

But it's a mistake to think that, in intimate relations, we can just relax and be appreciated for who we are (contra Govier 1998, p. 25). A normative notion of intimacy is not a retreat from moral struggle, where responsibility and accountability, self-reflection, repair, and forgiveness are part of the relationship landscape. The longed-for 'home' that Bearnice Johnson Reagon talks about, where one is barricaded from political and psychological struggles and where one goes to be revived and readied to return to the struggle elsewhere, should not be sought in intimate relations (Reagon 1983, p. 358). If we push too hard to find 'home' in intimacy, we are likely to impede the very closeness we seek. Genuine intimacy requires that we engage in moral struggle with our loved ones and with ourselves and, to be able to do that well, we need to be able to trust others and for others to trust us.

The very idea of home can become contaminated and scary for many women. The loss of home – or the inability to find and keep it – is a very real and tragic experience for some women and, coupled with cultural norms and expectations that are placed on women regarding relationships and family, can give rise to frustration, disappointment, self-blame, and rage. Longing for a place of acceptance without criticism, without challenge, and without fear of things going awry is an understandable but somewhat misguided desire; unconditional love and acceptance doesn't eliminate crises in relationships, misunderstandings, and moments of fear or accusation. And problems in relationships are not necessarily signs of a relationship in trouble. These are lessons that many BPD patients find hard to learn. A sense of belongingness, therefore, should not be equated with being home or at home, if by that we mean that home is a site without struggle. We can and should be able to feel we belong – in a relationship, in a family, in a church group – without having to avoid conflict or feel guilty when we must address conflict.

But consider that a search for home, in its ideal sense, can give rise to homesickness.

3.3.2 Homesickness, desperate love, and bisected beings

Between the seventeenth and nineteenth centuries, homesickness – then called nostalgia – was considered a medical condition with symptoms ranging from sadness, disturbed sleep, fluctuations in appetite, heart palpitations, diminished senses, dullness of mind, and a marked tendency to dwell solely on the past (Clarke 2007). Today, homesickness is usually thought of as psychological, but it can be physiological as well (cf. Thurber and Weisz 1997). Homesickness is tied to an ache for home and often is a problem found in immigrants and refugees who have left home. It is associated more strongly when the transition from home to the unfamiliar is perceived as outside one's control (Thurber and Weisz 1997).

Can we be homesick if we never had a home? Can we long for something we never had? The answer is yes, if we consider home and homesickness to be metaphors. In fact, the standard philosophical definition of desire is a longing for what one does not have. Desire is future oriented and contrastive: it moves us to try to fill a current lack rather than to reflect on satisfaction. It may be useful, in thinking about BPD women, to imaginatively engage in the concepts of home and homesickness as a search for the safety of home and the ache and longing for what they cannot find. Being without a home can make us sick.

Homesickness, in the sense I use it here, can create a feeling of desperation for home and love, and desperate love can give rise to fears of abandonment. Desperate love is characterized as:

> a feeling of fusion with the lover, an overwhelming desire for and anxiety concerning reciprocation, idealization of the lover, feelings of insecurity outside the relationship such that life is experienced as much more fulfilling when involved in the relationship, difficulty with interpersonal reality testing, and extremes of happiness and sadness.
>
> (Sperling 1985, p. 324)

The Desperate Love Scale, developed by Michael Sperling, measures such things as a feeling that a void is filled by being in the relationship. But identifying this feeling as that of desperation sits awkwardly in the light of over 2000 years of stories of romance. I recount just one.

In Plato's *Symposium*, for example, Aristophanes recounts the myth that we humans originally were beings of three kinds: male, female, and male-female. Furthermore, we were round, with four legs, four arms, two faces, two sets of genitals, and so on. Because we had eight limbs in all, we could get around very quickly and without tiring, thus threatening to surpass the gods. So, the gods decided to weaken us by cutting us in half.

> Now, when the work of bisection was complete it left each half with a desperate yearning for the other, and they ran together and flung their arms around each other's necks, and asked for nothing better than to be rolled into one. So much so, that they began to die of hunger and inertia, for neither would do anything without the other. And whenever one half was left alone by the death of its mate, it wandered about questing and clasping in the hope of finding a spare half-woman—or a whole woman, as we should call her nowadays—or half a man. And so the race was dying out.
>
> (Plato 1966, pp. 543–544)

To encourage reproduction, the gods moved the genitals to the front of the body. (Before this division, humans spilled their seed 'like grasshoppers,' but now, while we clung to one another, the seed could be deposited within the other.) While the *Symposium* was created in a different ethos and for a vastly different audience, many of the classics in the literature romanticize love – such as Charlotte Bronte's *Jane Eyre* (2006), where Jane has left Rochester after finding out that he is married, and then hears him calling her name, 'Jane, Jane' from many miles away; she rushes to him to discover his house and his wife have burned down and he is now blind but available. Some aspects of popular culture in the late twentieth century retain a form of this theme: many of us are searching for that 'kindred spirit,' that 'soulmate.'

For example, one young male, Peter, said of his relationship with Amy,

> Just being with somebody and knowing somebody just so well that, you know you can guess what they are thinking and what they are thinking all the time, it's just, yeah it's like, I feel like when we are together we are a whole person, when I am apart I am half a person.

(Allen 2003, p. 228)

It may be the silliness of a naive or romantic heart, but desperate love is fairly normalized in the western world. Intense, high-energy and all-absorbing romantic love often occurs at the beginning of a relationship but, as Leslie Greenberg and Rhonda Goldman (2008) point out, often is pathologized in psychotherapeutic circles. They argue that it should not be pathologized, at least early in a relationship: 'Merger exists at the beginning of any relationship: gay, lesbian, and heterosexual alike. It is typical to idealize partners, avoid disagreements, or feel bereft away from the relationship' (2008, p. 132). This is why I reframe such feelings in terms of a longing for belongingness and a misunderstanding of what home should consist in; the latter way doesn't medicalize longing and so avoids the connotation of psychopathology.

Let me summarize the argument. (Virtually) everyone, including BPD patients, needs to experience a sense of belonging, whether it is belonging with others, with a god, with a spirit world, or with nature. And even political activists who struggle daily with difference – like BPD patients who struggle with otherness (see Chapter 1) – long for home and feel homesick without it. So, the first point is that such longings and aims are neither unique to BPD patients nor *prima facie* signs of disturbance. Secondly, I have argued that it is a mistake to equate belongingness with a sense of home, if 'home' is conceptualized as a site without moral struggle, but that many, perhaps most, people do make this mistake. Being in relationship, whether political, psychological, or social, is not always safe and comfortable, and should not be strained to become so.

When the relationships of patients with BPD are rocky and tumultuous, they may in part indicate the sorts of moral struggle that Reagon says are vital to bringing about change. This is not to say that patients with BPD do not mishandle feelings of homesickness and desires for belongingness. They may indeed take desperate measures to avoid being abandoned; Sperling remarks that 'desperate love can be thought of as bearing resemblance to love relations typical of borderline character structure' (1985, p. 325). But – and this is the third point – homesickness and desperate love, whether it is felt by BPD patients or the rest of us, should not automatically be thought of as a medical condition, as it was in the past centuries, but as a longing for connectedness and belongingness that has been culturally approved since the time of Plato.

I suggest that homesickness comes in degrees. Paralyzing homesickness, where one is unable to leave home, creates problems that milder homesickness does not; desperate love, where one is unable to let go even in the face of violating the beloved's boundaries, leads to loss and grief that may have been avoided and, hence, is dysfunctional. BPD patients, because they lack earlier experiences of belongingness and connectedness, may have an especially difficult time navigating the difficult terrain of relationships where their desire for belongingness and desperation for love, their ambivalence about the safety of home, and their absence of skills for repairing damage that is done in relationships can exacerbate relational problems. Yet I remind readers that our conceptualizations of love, romance, relationships, intimacy, and belongingness are always embedded within a social and cultural context. Different cultures and different eras emphasize varying reasons for coupling, not just for romantic love and belongingness but also for utilitarian purposes or for protection or security. Rules for the expression of emotions such as love, sadness, and anger vary across cultures and genders and may make closeness more difficult for some (cf. Greenberg and Goldman 2008). And as women in most cultures are being encouraged (allowed?) to be more assertive and to expect equality in their relationships, it should come as no surprise that both traditional and non-traditional coupling can become rocky.

This concludes the framework within which I analyze BPD relationships. I now turn to research on gendered norms and expectations for relationships.

3.4 Relationship norms and expectations

As I discussed in Chapter 1, prevailing western theories of the self make normative claims about the eventual desirability of the mature adult to be autonomous and independent. But another standard of maturity is the ability to maintain stable and satisfying relationships; both independence and interdependence are, at least in theory, valued in western cultures. Yet gender stereotypes and gendered expectations of relationships may influence BPD women's anxiety and distrust about being in relationships. So, let me start by setting out some of the norms and expectations for relationships that studies have identified.

First, a caveat. Most of my data come from research done on heterosexual and, often, married couples, but I do not assume that either heterosexuality or marriage curtails the import of this section. Sally Duffy and Caryl Rusbult (1986) suggest that everyone, gay, lesbian, bisexual, or straight, is socialized in the same romantic heritage, a heritage that stresses monogamous involvement, romantic love, permanence, and so on. They found that, regardless of sexual orientation, women reported greater investment and greater commitment to maintain their relationships than did men.

Unrealistic expectations for relationships include ideas such as 'my partner should be able to read my mind and know what I need without my telling him or her' and 'my partner should always please me sexually'; assumptions about relationships such as that one's partner can't change, that disagreement is destructive, and that sexes are different are found to make coupling relationships dysfunctional (Foran and Slep 2007). It is, perhaps, obvious that unrealistic expectations and high standards can negatively affect relationships. Responses include blaming the partner, wanting to hurt the partner, and expressing negative affect such as anger (Foran and Slep 2007). Unrealistic expectations make it more difficult for conflicts to be resolved and make more difficult partners' ability to adapt to common marital stressors because they are rooted in irrational beliefs that impair one's ability to reason through things clearly. They make connection, mutual trust, and repair more difficult to cultivate.

Such relationship difficulties plague both men and women. But evidence abounds that expectations and assumptions are different for different genders.

Nuray Sakalli-Ugurlu examined (heterosexual romantic) relationship satisfaction, as measured by commitment, rewards and costs of the relationship, stability of the relationship, perceived alternatives to the relationship, time spent together, power sharing, and future time orientation (2003, p. 295). Future time orientation in romantic relationships (FTORR) is a skill set and schema of the person's ability to foresee, form expectations about, and plan for the future (p. 295), and earlier studies suggested that more future time oriented people are less satisfied with their relationships. Sakalli-Ugurlu found that women are more future oriented than are men, have more future plans for relationships and family, work harder to maintain relationships, and are significantly more committed to romantic relationships (cf. Nurmi 1991; Sacher and Fine 1996). And while both men and women believe that marking special occasions (with a card, flowers, etc.) is an important sign of love, women are found to place greater emphasis on mutual activity, offerings, selflessness (doing favors for the other; helping the other with problems), and willingness to make sacrifices for the partner (Lemieux 1996).

Paul Amato *et al.* (2007) extensively compared marriages in 1980 and 2000. They report that changes in the cultural climate of marriage make them more unstable, even though many changes (such as fewer patriarchal marriages and the freedom to leave unequal relationships) are positive.

> Despite these potential benefits, growing support for nontraditional gender arrangements in marriage is likely to clash with the existing gender-based division of labor and the patriarchal power relations that continue to underpin many marriages.
>
> (Amato *et al.* 2007, p. 27)

Women have more readily embraced non-traditional ideas about marriage and gender roles, giving rise to conflicting expectations between husbands and wives (p. 27). For example, wives' expectations that their husbands will share in the housework if both are working full-time do not appear to be met. Even though husbands report doing more housework in 2000 than in 1980, they often are not perceived as doing an equal share, which perceptions of unfairness contribute to resentment and arguments (p. 28). Arlie Hochschild in 1989 reported that many employed wives come home to do what she termed the 'second shift' of cooking dinner, washing dishes, and doing housekeeping chores; Amato *et al.* found that 32% of wives report doing a second shift still in 2000 (2007, p. 157). While this is an improvement, it doesn't lessen the likelihood that many wives working both outside and inside the home will feel resentment at husbands who do not seem to treat housework equally. Perceived unfairness leads to lower marital quality, and wives reported less happiness, less interaction, more conflict, more problems, and greater divorce proneness; in other words, wives come out in both 1980 and in 2000 as experiencing lower marital quality in all five dimensions (Amato *et al.* 2007, p. 211).

Another change Amato *et al.* reported is that couples' decision-making has shifted from patriarchal (husband almost always has the final say) to a more equal model, a dimension that wives relate more strongly to marital quality than do husbands (p. 220). Women in relationships where they feel that they do not have a voice or are not consulted about decisions affecting both of them may feel angry, even furious, if they have come to adopt newer norms for marriage and coupling relationships; expectations of fairness and equality may clash with her partner's more traditional expectations. These points hark back to earlier chapter discussions about double binds for women as they try to fit changing and conflicting cultural norms for femaleness – independent, income-earner, nurturer, homemaker, housekeeper, good mother, wife and lover, and sane to boot!

If these findings hold true, then they can account for some of the rockiness and disappointment that female BPD patients report about their (heterosexual romantic) relationships. Yet questions remain. Do these changes in relationship satisfaction correlate to an increase in the BPD diagnosis? Are BPD patients' relationships any less volatile because cultural reasons for women's dissatisfaction exist? Are we pathologizing volatility where we should not? It still may be true, in many cases, that the way women express their dissatisfaction is counterproductive in the long run. Think back to the Walkers: Jacqueline got what she wanted but at the cost of her husband's resentment and only by portraying herself as helpless to take care of herself for a short time. Therapeutic intervention may, therefore, be very useful even if we don't consider desperate measures to be symptomatic of mental disorder.

3.5 Critiques of norms and expectations as they relate to BPD

For women in most parts of the world, the clinical picture of psychological health and academic theories of moral psychology combine to reinforce norms for relationship that are detrimental to women. Empirical evidence that women hold higher expectations than men do and greater difficulty feeling satisfied in relationships fits into theories of relationship where women are *supposed* to do the primary relationship work. This section is meant to illustrate how women's longing for belongingness, home, trust, and connected relationships can collide with entrenched cultural norms that valorize being in relationships and doing relationship work, particularly for women.

Kant's and Mill's moral theories, the prevailing ones from the modern period until now, emphasized universal principles, the rights of the individual, and fairness or justice. Each theory offers a systematic, deductive, and logical method for determining what the right thing to do is. These theories have been dubbed, together, the ethic of justice; they offer a moral psychology where reason, in order to attain morality and autonomy, must not be tainted by emotion or attachments (cf. Kant 1993b; Mill 2002). The ethic of justice contrasts with the 'ethic of care.' The ethic of care was identified as a 'different voice' by Carol Gilligan (1982), who argued that the moral reasoning of women is based on values of attachment, relationship, and inclusiveness. She argues that women reason from within the context of relationships rather than universally and abstractly. Gilligan and other researchers (Bornstein *et al.* 2004) give empirical grounding to the long-held popular belief that women are 'better at relationships' than are men (cf. Gray 1992; Ruddick 1983; Noddings 1984). The idea, both in academia and in popular culture, is that men are more autonomous and independent while women are more interdependent. This idea gave rise to such self-help books as *Men are from Mars, Women are from Venus* (Gray 1992) and *You just don't understand: Women and men in conversation* (Tannen 2001), books that essentialize gender differences (meaning that those authors believe that gender differences in communication and valuing of relationships are biological). According to Gilligan, women think of themselves as selves-in-relation and, on this view, thinking about themselves that way is a good thing: men and women conceptualize themselves differently and reason about morality differently, but nevertheless both conceptions and styles of reasoning are valuable (Claudia Card calls this the 'rosy view'; (Card 1990, p. 202)). Even though some women are not particularly good at sustaining intimate relationships, most women come to believe that their development requires intimacy and connection and that meaningfulness will (or should) arise out of relationships. Thus, an emphasis on sustaining attachment and connection can intersect with gendered ideas about women and relationships in ways that may cloud our understanding of BPD.

3.5.1 The 'female ethic' overly burdens women

If women are expected to be better at relationships – and more invested in them – they are expected to do more of the relationship work, what Elizabeth Spelman calls 'relationship repair' (Spelman 2004). According to her, 'the household … is designated as the default location for people to fuel up and get washed, clothed, and reclothed; it's where they're to receive the daily doses of repair and restoration necessary for them to keep on going, physically, mentally, and emotionally …' (p. 47). And women are (still) the primary people who do this repair work in the household, much of which is relationship repair. Because of this, Spelman suggests that an ethic of care is a more useful moral theory for what needs to be done in the home than the ethic of justice because the ethic of care understands morality to be about relationships, not about principles. Relationships break down, they strain, they get muddled, and they get enmeshed, and relationship- and self-repair are necessary for us to continue with our lives.

I am reluctant to endorse Spelman's claim that an ethic of care is better than other moral theories as a way to conceptualize relational repair because of its essentializing aspects for females. The view that women are especially good at relationships burdens women. As we saw in the first half of this chapter, whether as mothers, daughters, friends, wives, or female partners, women are socialized to expect that they should do most of the repair that is needed; men are socialized to expect the women in their lives to 'naturally' be better at nurturing, connecting, and sustaining relationships. Furthermore, other kinds of repair – car repair, household appliances – can be outsourced; relationship repair cannot. And women who cannot, or will not, do relationship repair are judged as lacking in womanly characteristics.

3.5.2 Aretha and the 'natural woman' problem

Similarly, women, who either are not interested in relationships or are not very good at them, are judged as flawed women. Some women, like some men, are independent, some are loners, some enjoy socializing but not intimacy, and some are bad at relationships. It's an open question whether or not a person who is a loner, or independent, has formed some underlying psychological weakness or undergone a trauma that impedes sociality (cf. Krakauer's *Into the Wild* (2007)). Nevertheless, cultural norms for femaleness include the idea that women have a greater need for connection and closeness than do men. Again, those who fall short of norms for womanhood – who fall outside the essence of woman as described by popular culture and academia alike – are considered less than fully women.

3.5.3 Attachment valorized

Finally, I consider the conceptual and moral problem of praising women for their 'natural' commitment to attachments by drawing on Claudia Card's work. Being attached isn't unequivocally good, and to think so is to romanticize attachment and relationality (Card 1990, p. 202). Women are socialized to value ideals of love, loyalty, and forgiveness and they internalize the expectation that women in particular long for connection. These norms may lead women who are in debilitating relationships to minimize trouble and suppress danger and harm. 'Not every passionate attachment to persons is valuable, any more than every passionate espousal of principles is. The nature and basis of the attachment matters' (Card 1990, p. 215).

A single-minded commitment to a bad relationship reflects bad judgment. But it also reflects bad moral luck. Moral luck is the kind of chance occurrence outside our control that affects whether or not we are responsible for good or bad consequences (cf. Williams 1976, Nagel 1979). Bad luck that is gendered is luck that socializes virtues of relationship and personal attachment that are harmful to women. Since gender expectations place a greater burden on women to stay in bad relationships in order to be 'good,' this is a sign of moral bad luck. Card argues that framing attachment as a 'women's virtue' reifies attachment and does not encourage women to distinguish between good and bad attachments. This cognitive skill would seem to be both morally and psychologically necessary for BPD patients to develop. It is also crucial to take into account that relationship difficulties are not only psychiatric kinds but are cultural, social, and reasoning ones: ambivalence, ambiguity, and contradiction are not easily countenanced in Western societies.

3.6 **Conclusion**

My interest in this chapter is in the normative force of these ideas in shaping assessments of women and potential pathological symptoms. If mature, healthy women are (normatively) expected to form and value attachments, relationality, and connectedness, does this expectation cloud clinicians' judgments when they perceive women who do not conform to the norm? Are women who present with unstable interpersonal relationships more likely to be viewed as pathologically relationally troubled? I suggest that the norms of womanhood influence how we view women's relationship troubles, but clinical studies will be necessary to address this question (cf. Flanagan and Blashfield 2003; Linehan 1993).

I also suggest that a complementary way to the DSMs in thinking about women in tumultuous relationships is to focus on trust and betrayal, home and homesickness, and connection and repair. In sorting out what counts as a healthy relationship and what counts as a pathological one, we need to examine how the formation of early betrayal along with a need for connection leads to vacillating attitudes toward those the BPD patient wants to trust. Thus, clinicians need to develop an ethic of trustworthiness that allows for patients to learn that it is sometimes safe to trust another. Trust and trustworthiness are so central to patient recovery from BPD, and so difficult to navigate given entrenched distrust, that I devote a chapter to the ethic of trustworthiness in Part II of this book. Finally, because emotions are one of the most culturally embedded aspects of our inner world and because the rules and reasons for forming relationships are cultural (Greenberg and Goldman 2008), we must treat people in their particularity and their local contexts and not as abstract or representational entities.

Chapter 4

Impulsivity, spontaneity, and deliberation

4.1 **An example**

Rachel, a mother of two who eventually gets diagnosed with BPD, is arguing with her husband Tim. It is evening time. As Rachel's anger and accusations escalate, she sees Tim becoming desperate and impatient with her. 'No, not again, Rachel. Don't do this again. I can't take anymore of it!'

> That clinched it. He hated me. He'd leave me, broke, with these two little kids and the piece of shit house. No, no! He couldn't leave me. I wouldn't give the son of a bitch the satisfaction.
>
> The tears halted immediately, and I felt a rush of energy. Barefoot, in gym shorts, without so much as grabbing the car keys, I ran out the door and down the alley. I could hear Tim pleading with me to come back and frantically apologizing for losing his patience. I felt power rising within me. I didn't look back and kept on going.
>
> I didn't have a destination in mind, but as I kept jogging down the streets of the city, I realized I was heading to the West Side. If I were lucky, I'd make it to the projects. If I were even luckier, the God I didn't really believe existed would have mercy on me and let me become just another crime statistic. Suicide roulette. I ran for miles, barefoot and westward through the glass-strewn sidewalks of declining neighborhoods.

(Reiland 2004, pp. 16–17)

Is Rachel being impulsive by going on a run in the evening? It doesn't seem to have been planned because she was barefoot and didn't know where she was heading. The run seems to have been risky behavior in that she knowingly placed herself in danger. But why identify Rachel's behavior as impulsive, rather than spontaneous? What would it take for her to do something different from going on this nighttime run as a result of her argument with Tim? And what is gained and what is lost if she avoids this run?

4.2 **Constructs in need of conceptual analysis**

Clinicians – and the public in general – view impulsive behavior as dysfunctional. With respect to BPD, impulsivity is arguably one of the core behavioral symptoms. We generally assume that people won't engage in self-destructive actions if they can help it, and deliberation is assumed to prevent self-destructive actions. Impulsivity is of concern because some patients' actions are self-destructive, undermining their attempts at improvement. Studies also suggest that impulsive behavior is linked to affective instability (cf. Gunderson 2001, pp. 41–44; but note that this combination can be found both in BPD patients and in ones diagnosed with bipolar disorder). Impulsive behavior plus mood swings can wreak havoc on interpersonal relationships, so these behaviors must be examined in the light of their consequences to the BPD patient. Nevertheless, the concept of impulsivity is unclear, and thus its application in evaluating behavior is sometimes problematic.

Impulsive behavior is thought to be the antithesis of deliberative behavior. In western philosophy, actions that are performed based on a good reasoning process are the hallmark of the rational person. Deliberation is praiseworthy, when done well, and the actions that follow (including a decision not to act) are chosen because they advance a person's goals and projects, or they are anticipated to contribute to living a flourishing life. Although both impulsivity and spontaneity are thought to be 'in-the-moment' behaviors, impulsive behavior is viewed as negative while spontaneous behavior typically is praised. (Later, I will explain the complication that many behaviors described as impulsive seem to be planned out).

About impulsivity, Marsha Linehan writes that 'suicidal and other impulsive, dysfunctional behaviors are usually maladaptive solution behaviors to the problem of overwhelming, uncontrollable, intensely painful negative affect' (Linehan 1993, p. 60). Spontaneity, by contrast, seems to be good: some philosophers argue that spontaneity is a necessary aspect of freedom (cf. Glenn 1980). Other philosophers argue that it is vital to the creative process (for example, for jazz musicians; cf. Brown 2000, 1996). Some virtue theorists argue that spontaneity is important to good character (cf. Walker 1992; Digby 1980). Deliberation about action would seem to undermine spontaneity (which would be a loss, presumably), but it would also undermine impulsivity (which presumably would be a good thing).

In 4.3, I give an overview of clinical definitions of impulsivity. In 4.4 and 4.5, I unpack the reasoning that is involved in deliberative and impulsive behavior. I apply these concepts to the example of Rachel, above, and to Maggie, who repeatedly cuts herself. In 4.6, I analyze spontaneous behavior by drawing on jazz and suggest what is valuable about being spontaneous. In 4.7, I consider one kind of activity that is associated with impulsivity in BPD, casual sex, with the aim of clarifying the values and assumptions that underlie moral evaluations of casual sex. In particular, I argue that women are evaluated differently than men when it comes to sex behaviors and that a gender bias may influence whether clinicians view women who engage in casual sex as symptomatic of BPD. Finally, I introduce the Olaf principle as a possible way to distinguish between spontaneity and impulsivity. The significance of the Olaf principle is that it offers a way to distinguish between the two without resorting to appraisal by others, thus potentially avoiding the importation of moral values in understanding impulsivity. Although I believe that impulsivity and spontaneity are more on a continuum than distinct categories, the Olaf principle, in conjunction with an analysis of impulsivity and spontaneity, can help us understand when and why impulsivity is symptomatic of a mental disorder.

4.3 **Clinical definitions of impulsivity**

Impulsivity is a characteristic associated with a number of mental disorders, such as BPD and antisocial personality disorder (APD), attention-deficit/hyperactivity disorder, mania, and substance-related disorders (Dowson *et al.* 2004, p. 29). In patients with BPD, the criterion of impulsivity evolved out of the literature that called attention to 'acting out as a resistance to, or flight from, feelings or conflicts' (Gunderson 2001, p. 9). Gunderson notes both that one pattern of impulsivity can be substituted for another and that impulsivity is a temperament (2001, p. 10). By calling something a temperament, one identifies that behavior pattern as biophysiological and, therefore, hard-wired. Fehon *et al.* report that '"the presence of PTSD symptomatology and the trait of impulsivity in particular play a more important role" in the overall prediction of violent behavior. As such, the psychiatric sequelae of childhood trauma, namely the development of PTSD and its characteristic features of emotional and behavioral dysregulation, hyperreactivity, and sensitivity, may predispose traumatized youth toward impulsive behaviors such as violence and aggression' (Fehon *et al.* 2005, p. 410).

Dowson *et al.* state that impulsive behaviors involve 'relatively unpremeditated aggressive behavior directed to self or others in the context of BPD or APD' (2004, p. 29). Moeller *et al.* (2001) define impulsivity as 'a predisposition toward rapid, unplanned reactions to internal or external stimuli without regard to the negative consequences of these reactions to the impulsive individual or to others.' Other behaviors under this rubric 'have included acting without thinking about negative consequences; a rapid emotional response involving impatience, irritability, anger, or aggression; and taking undue risks' (Dowson *et al.* 2004, p. 29).

John Evenden gives as examples of impulsive behavior 'taking one more drink, an extra purchase at the supermarket or just stopping and chatting to a friend met unexpectedly in the street' (Evenden 1999a, p. 348). But Evenden says that impulsivity is part of everyday life that adds color to ordinary experience. He rightly notes that considerable disagreement exists as to how to distinguish socially acceptable impulsive behavior from dysfunctional (1999a, p..348). By including activities such as stopping to chat with a friend in the concept of impulsivity and by saying that impulsivity adds color to our lives, Evenden seems to collapse impulsivity and spontaneity. I am sympathetic to that move, but it ultimately fails to clarify what genuinely is troubling about some BPD impulsive behavior – in particular, repeated self-injurious behavior (see Chapter 5).

A literature review by Evenden (1999b) discusses the various definitions of impulsivity and disagreement about what sorts of behaviors are included in the construct. Evenden identifies two common themes: one refers to 'a tendency to fail to analyse and reflect before engaging in a behaviour, and the second refers to consideration of the results of the behavior, perhaps even preferring a risky outcome' (1999b, p. 181). But, as I will argue, neither of these themes quite hits the mark for the construct of impulsivity. Although a tendency to be deliberative before acting is a good thing, we shouldn't *always* analyze and reflect before engaging in behavior: all rational self-reflection and non-spontaneous behavior makes Jill a dull girl. And although it is usually valuable to consider the consequences before we act, there is no obvious reason why we shouldn't sometimes take risks for a chance of a highly valued outcome that couldn't be achieved any other way. (For instance, a risky investment that has a chance of producing a high return might, in the context of an otherwise well-balanced portfolio, be a more reasonable choice than a lower-risk investment with a high probability of a low return).

Readers may notice that impulsive behavior is not unique to BPD. Furthermore, nearly all other criteria help diagnosticians distinguish BPD from other mental disorders. So getting clear on just what impulsivity is may not help us to understand how impulsivity relates specifically to BPD patients. Therefore, although I can clarify the central constructs and underlying values dwelling within impulsivity, I am conservative regarding its usefulness in application to BPD.

4.4 **Deliberation**

The emphasis placed on deliberation goes all the way back to ancient times, where the ideal of human excellence requires that our actions reflect a life plan. The idea is that our choices should be structured so that our various goals and projects are ordered toward an ultimate end. The ultimate end should capture our idea about what it is for a human to flourish (Cooper 1975, pp. 16–18). This means that our immediate decisions are always situated in the context of planning for the future, and our plans for the future impact our choices now (Sherman 1989, p. 74). To deliberate is to work through a process of what to do or not do, given one's values, beliefs, aims, and facts of the situation (Cooper 1975, p. 5). Deliberation contains our reasons for acting, and so we can appeal to those reasons when asked why we chose to do what we did (Cooper 1975, p. 9). This point is important in thinking about Rachel's late-night run: if Rachel can't answer the question, 'Why did you go on that risky run and without shoes?' then she doesn't have a reason for that behavior, according to Cooper and, without reasons, her action of going on that run cannot be said to be the result of deliberation. But it is not necessarily the case that if deliberation did not lead to this run, Rachel was acting impulsively. We do things out of habit, and we do things that we already decided upon long ago (for example, if I'm a Kantian, I don't ever need to deliberate about whether or not to lie because lying is always wrong to do. So, that issue is forever settled). At any rate, Rachel does seem to be able to give an answer: she isn't saying, 'Gosh I don't know why I did that.' She explains that she is feeling punitive. So, the issue may not be that she didn't deliberate but that her deliberation led to what we might consider a poor conclusion. Having reasons and having good reasons are two different things. So, we need to dig deeper into another quality of deliberation – that thinking about what we should do should be set within the larger context of goals and aims for our lives. Note that I now have introduced a second kind of deliberation – the kind that is broad and takes into account what sorts of actions will bring about our flourishing in the long run. This is a norm of deliberation that may be relevant particularly in cases of BPD actions, a topic I return to in 4.6.

Let me say more about norms of reasoning. Good deliberation requires that we have experience of persons and situations others have lived through (Sherman 1989, p. 48), that we have capacities for reasoning and inferring, and that we have enough concrete information about *this* situation so that we don't have to investigate further. If we lack such information, we must investigate first and deliberate later.

Being able to deliberate well in the broad sense means making choices that add up to flourishing, both for ourselves and for others. Good deliberation is crucial because the choices we make indicate the sort of person we are, and the quality and content of our character makes some choices more attractive, others less. To quote Aristotle, 'For in fact we are ourselves in a way jointly responsible for our states of character, and the sort of character we have determines the sort of end [aim or goal] we lay down' (Aristotle 1999, 1114b22–1114b25). This view of the relation between character and choice places quite a bit of responsibility in our own hands for who we become. One question, then, is whether or not we should excuse BPD patients for their impulsive behavior on the grounds that they cannot help what they do (they are ill, personality disordered) or whether, instead, we should blame them for becoming the sort of person who fails to deliberate. The larger problem, as we have seen in earlier chapters, is that it looks like patients are blamed for 'bad' actions, where blame entails that the agent could have done otherwise. But if blame is appropriate for BPD patients' 'bad' actions, then it is not clear that we are dealing with a psychiatric kind: it is inconsistent to blame someone for things they do as a result of their illness. I take up this issue more directly in Chapter 6, where I investigate the charge of BPD patients' manipulative behaviors.

Good reasoners are not merely rational calculators. Deliberation also employs the use of emotions. Emotions, properly educated, can help us see more clearly what we are facing in the moment and what sorts of attitudes and actions are called for. As Nancy Sherman says, '... without emotions, we do not fully register the facts or record them with the sort of resonance and importance that only emotional involvement can sustain" (1989, p. 47). Like Iris Murdoch (1970), Sherman uses the metaphor of 'seeing' to explain the role of emotion in deliberation: seeing through emotions provides a platform of supportive motives that help us be moved to the action that we intellectually recognize as the right one (1989, p. 48). Alison Jaggar argues (1989) that emotions are epistemologically significant, meaning that they give us knowledge we might otherwise miss (cf. also Stocker 1976). The person who has trouble with emotion regulation may also have trouble with the broad sense of deliberation because, as her moods swiftly change, her perceptions are colored accordingly.

In philosophy, we recognize a problem of knowing the correct or morally right thing to do, and then failing to do that action. This problem, identified as *akrasia* by Aristotle, is commonly called weakness of the will. As Martha Nussbaum sets it out (2001), the reasoning goes like this:

> A must choose between x and y.
> A knows that x is better or preferable to y.
> A chooses y.

This requires explanation: how could a rational being knowingly choose the inferior or worse thing? Plato's answer is that we don't – no one chooses the bad knowingly. His reasoning is that, although choice x is objectively better than choice y, I may, from my subjective judgment, think y is better and so choose y. This is a mistake in judgment that I make because I am ignorant of what the features of choice x really are. According to Plato, this is why someone would do something bad.

Aristotle's answer is to develop a complex explanation of two kinds of knowing, one where someone has it without using it and another where someone has it and uses it. Aristotle explains that the *akratic* person draws the correct conclusion but fails to activate it or attend to it (Aristotle 1999, 1146b30–1147a15). Then, passions override reason.

It is tempting to explain Rachel's risky late-night run in terms of *akrasia*: if she takes time to think about it, considering the time of day, her sports clothing needs, the location of a run, her safety, and the worry she would cause her family if she were to go on a night run, barefoot, in the projects, surely she would not go on that run. But she 'knows' all that, and she goes on the run anyway. Her passion overrides her better judgment.

But old-fashioned weakness of the will may not apply here. According to Amélie Rorty, the *akratic* person is capable of intentional action, normal and relatively fine sensory discrimination, and constitutionally capable of acting and reacting within a mean; she has intellectual virtues and can make proper inferences (Rorty 1980, p. 271). It's an open question whether or not patients with BPD have these cognitive capacities. If they do not, then their impulsivity wouldn't come under this rubric because weakness of the will is blameworthy and lacking cognitive skills for deliberation is not blameworthy. If BPD patients do have such cognitive capacities and skills, then it might be appropriate to think of impulsivity as a kind of *akrasia*, but then we run into another problem, as I alluded to earlier: impulsivity would be a moral kind and, perhaps, not a psychiatric kind (cf. Zachar and Potter forthcoming).

4.5 **Impulsivity and willing[1]**

Bernard Gert and Timothy Duggan (1979) provide an insightful analysis of willing that will serve as my starting point in understanding the problem of impulsivity. Their account of free will combines the idea of having the ability to will with the idea of voluntary mental or physical ability. The emphasis on 'ability' highlights the point that abilities are usually 'relatively enduring properties of persons' (Gert and Duggan 1979, p. 199). 'Willing,' according to Gert and Duggan, is 'doing intentionally or trying to do' (1979, p. 216n5) – but it is the ability to will kinds of actions that distinguish those acts for which we are responsible and those for which we are not.

According to Gert and Duggan, the ability to will is tied to the ability to believe that what I will call conclusive reasons exist not to do a particular act

---

[1] Impulsivity can be contrasted with careful planning, due consideration, and generally dependable and predictable actions.

of kind x.[2] 'A [conclusive reason] is one which it would be unreasonable to expect *any* rational person not to act on' (Gert and Duggan 1979, p. 203; emphasis in original). A conclusive reason is a trump in deliberation. There exist two ways to lack the ability to will to do actions of kind x. One is when a person believes something irrational and no evidence to the contrary can convince him otherwise. Gert and Duggan give the example of someone who believes that he must visit his mother's grave every Sunday or something terrible will happen, and he cannot be persuaded otherwise. A conclusive reason might be if he believed that he would, perhaps irrevocably, alienate his wife by refusing to spend some Sundays at family events. The authors conclude that since this man doesn't have the ability to believe that conclusive reasons exist that could get him to do otherwise, he lacks the ability to will not to visit the grave.

The other example Gert and Duggan give is of someone who compulsively washes his hands every hour: he knows that he has conclusive reasons to refrain from hourly hand washing (the skin on his hands is sloughing off from frequent and harsh washing), but he does not act from these incentives (1979, p. 204). This person acts intentionally but not voluntarily – he lacks the ability to will not to wash his hands, even though he wills the action (in the sense of intending it) and, hence, cannot be said to be responsible for such actions. They categorize such actions as 'unvoluntary' to distinguish them from intentional but voluntary ones.

Unvoluntary actions, according to Gert and Duggan, exhibit a 'disability of the will' or 'volitional disability' (1979, p. 206). These are actions caused by 'something within the agent,' a dysfunction of the will regarding certain kinds of action. As Gert and Duggan rightly note, philosophy ignored this category for over 2000 years, with the consequence that it obscures our understanding of some forms of mental illness (1979, p. 212). 'The category of unvoluntary acts has a special relationship to mental illness. Indeed, to suffer a disability of the will is to suffer one form of mental illness ...' (1979, p. 213).

Let's apply this picture of unvoluntary action to a BPD patient, Maggie. Maggie regularly shows up in the emergency room after cutting herself. Now in one sense she did it intentionally, in that she intended that action. She had to do at least some planning: she had to find an instrument with which to cut herself, she had to find a room in which to do it, and she had to choose a site on her body (an example that suggests that it is a mistake to think that impulsivity

---

[2] Gert and Duggan's term is 'coercive incentives' but that phrase is too laden with philosophical complexity for my purposes. Also, I'm slightly simplifying Gert and Duggan's account by paying less attention to non-coercive incentives because I don't think the full theory makes a significant difference to this analysis.

only is sudden or 'in the moment'). Is Maggie exhibiting a volitional disorder when it comes to self-injurious behavior?

One way we might understand Maggie's cutting as unvoluntary is if she believes that cutting herself will relieve her tension and nothing within her belief set would make her change her mind. No conclusive reason within her belief system exists. For example, she doesn't believe that her father will get angry with her (although he will) because he has to pay the bills when she needs stitches; she doesn't believe her therapist will discontinue therapy if she cuts again (although her therapist has said so). Thus, according to Gert and Duggan's analysis of willing, Maggie lacks the ability to will not to cut herself. Therefore, when she does cut herself, she is not doing so freely but rather unvoluntarily. This could be one meaning of impulsive behavior, then; these are kinds of actions that one 'can't help' but do because something is faulty within the patient's belief system. Alternatively, as with the compulsive hand washer, Maggie might well believe that there exist conclusive reasons for her not to cut – she might indeed believe her therapist will terminate therapy, and she does not want that consequence – but she cannot get her belief system to motivate her to the better action. Here something between belief and motivation has broken down, the second kind of problem of the will.

Gert and Duggan's work is important for its contribution to a little-theorized area of action and willing, where the person does a kind of action intentionally but seems not to be free to will that kind of action, in any robust sense of willing. The typical philosophical divide has been between actions freely done and actions coerced by external forces. Gert and Duggan's theory opens the door to thinking about what we might call internal coercion, where what goes wrong in willing occurs internally. And it is distinct from *akrasia* in that it isn't cast as a moral failing. But their emphasis on the ability to believe as the core component of the ability to will leaves out a concept that others, myself included, think is central to the freedom to will – that of desire.

Another account of willing comes from Wright Neely (1974). While Neely would agree with Gert and Duggan that intentional actions are explained partly by reference to the agent's beliefs, he focuses on the role of desires in ascertaining whether a particular action is freely done. His notion of 'desire' includes whims, primary appetites, enduring character traits, and moral convictions. Freedom is more than just doing what one wants to do because, he argues, one can have an irresistible desire; being free requires that we 'have something to say about what we desire' (Neely 1974, p. 37). Neely's account of free desire acknowledges that we often (all of us) have incompatible desires, and thus he states that:

> A man is free to the extent that he does as he pleases provided that he can do otherwise (at least in the sense that if he did not want to be doing what he is doing, he

would not be doing it), and provided that (and to the extent that) he is not, in doing as he pleases, frustrating his ability to achieve other things that he desires to achieve.

(Neely 1974, p. 40)

We can make choices about which desires to pursue in the face of conflict by prioritizing them. Neely explains this prioritizing as follows: 'an agent's desire that-p is of higher priority than his desire that-q if and only if he desires that *if he must choose between satisfying his desire that-p and satisfying his desire that-*q, *he will satisfy his desire that-*p' (1974, p. 44; emphasis in original). These 'higher order' desires are more intimately tied to the self. Now, we can make sense of free action even while we acknowledge that we nearly always have conflicting desires. 'A man is freer to the extent that the desires out of which he acts are of relatively high priority as compared with those desires which conflict with them' (Neely 1974, p. 45).

Let's see how this theory might help in understanding what impulsivity is. Neely frames volitional disorders in terms of irresistible desires. He argues that 'a desire is irresistible if and only if it is the case that if the agent had been presented with *what he took to be* good and sufficient reason for not acting on it, he would still have acted on it' (1974, p. 47; emphasis in original). Suppose Maggie has been in therapy long enough to identify a higher order desire not to cut herself and an additional higher order desire not to distress her family and therapist by cutting. If these desires genuinely are hers, then even if Maggie still has a desire to cut herself, she also has what she takes to be good reasons not to do so. If she still cuts, despite her identified priorities, she might be said to have an irresistible desire.

Alfred Mele (2005) thinks Neely's account of irresistible desires is so demanding that almost nothing will count as irresistible. The worry is that we can imagine a situation that gives a strong enough reason for someone to resist a desire that is very, very hard to resist – for example, if you put a gun to that person's head. Mele argues that what makes a desire irresistible is whether or not, *at the time of action*, that person could have resisted doing that action but did not. But what is relevant in judging irresistibility is the desires and reasons now, in this situation, not the desires and reasons in a thought experiment. Mele questions whether volitional disorders should be cashed out in terms of irresistible desires, on the grounds that some people with volitional disorders might have desires that are very hard to resist but nevertheless are resistible. He draws upon Carl Elliott, who says that 'Often, a person suffering from a volitional disorder "is faced with the choice between (1) acting on desires that he finds morally repellent and shameful, and (2) refraining, which causes him considerable distress"' (Mele 2005, p. 81). If Mele is right, a genuinely irresistible desire is a compulsion, while a volitional disorder is one where actions are 'chosen' in a limited sense of the word. A desire to go on a night run, or to cut oneself, then, might be seen as something very very hard to resist but resistable so that when Rachel goes on that run, or Maggie cuts herself, the action is chosen in the sense that she could have done otherwise. If volitional disorders can explain impulsivity, then impulsivity is not fully unvoluntary in Gert and Duggan's sense.[3]

But this seems to present a different problem – namely, that it requires that, in order for one to have a volitional disorder, one has to be critically reflective, have higher order desires, and so on. So, if this idea applies to impulsivity, no actions will count as impulsive if we don't have a life plan, or at least some desires that, in theory, are in a position to be overridden by others. I think we can retain the idea of volitional disorders in the case of BPD since most patients do have some cognitive capacity for critical reflection and some of both first- and second-order desires.[4] But this discussion harks back to the problem that deliberation, as it is generally understood, requires us to be overly rational and that, as we saw with Evenden, impulsive behavior is described as actions that one has failed fully to consider. Furthermore, the analysis of unvoluntary actions and that of volitional disorders leaves open the possibility that one can fully consider the consequences of an action and yet not be moved to choose that action. Both the notion of deliberation and that of impulsivity set the bar so high that the ideal human is a thinking machine. And that picture seems to miss something important about the value of spontaneity.

4.6 **Spontaneity and the good life**

Let's now see if we can situate spontaneity in relation to impulsivity and deliberation. I'll begin with spontaneity. Why are one kind of actions – impulsive ones – considered bad while another kind of actions – spontaneous ones – are considered good when neither seems to involve deliberation and well-thought-through choosing? Daruna and Barnes seem to wonder about the same thing:

> The term impulsivity is usually reserved for maladaptive behaviour. The behavioural universe thought to reflect impulsivity encompasses actions that appear poorly

---

[3] What we have, so far, is that impulsivity is a partly unvoluntary kind of action that exhibits a volitional disorder. We can retain the idea that an impulsive person has higher order desires not to do what she does, in fact, end up doing. A volitional disorder, then, is a dysfunction of the will regarding some kind of action and in the context of a larger view of life-goals that order the person's desires but that the person is (unvoluntarily) unable to be guided by. So, we can see one reason why such actions are normatively bad: they unvoluntarily go against one's own larger scope plans.

[4] Since this book went to press, I have expanded on the volition-based versus non-volitional accounts of moral responsibility and blame in Zachar and Potter 2009b, forthcoming.

conceived, prematurely expressed, unduly risky, or inappropriate to the situation and that often result in undesirable consequences. When such actions have positive outcomes, they tend not to be seen as signs of impulsivity, but as indicators of boldness, quickness, spontaneity, courageousness, or unconventionality.

(Daruna and Barnes 1993, as quoted in Evenden 1999b)

I have already noted that it is incorrect to conceive of impulsivity as only 'in the moment' actions. Many actions that would be considered unvoluntary and to involve irresistible desires still involve some planning and preparation. (Rachel's run is more impulsive than Maggie's cutting, on that view, although both involve risky behavior, because Maggie at least had to do some planning before cutting, whereas Rachel didn't change into running clothes, put on running shoes, choose a route, etc).

To investigate differences between impulsivity and spontaneity and to uncover normative differences, I turn to jazz music. I admit this is an unusual choice; my reason for drawing on jazz is simply that this venue provides the best discussion and analysis of the value of spontaneity that I could find.

Lee Brown (1996), in theorizing differences between jazz and other modes of music that follow identifiable and expectable patterns, argues that jazz necessarily does not (and indeed cannot and still properly be called 'jazz') follow the 'principle of continuity.' Jazz is improvisational, by which is meant that the musician 'makes substantive decisions about what music to play *while* playing it' (1996, p. 354; emphasis in original). It is non-repeatable, flexible, and searching (Brown 1996, pp. 361–362 and p. 365).

Brown writes that, '[w]hile, for the sake of economy, I shall often speak of improvisers as creating music spontaneously, the hyperbole is not intended to rule it out that an improviser's decisions while playing are often guided by a larger conception of where he or she is going' (1996, p. 354), such as normative elements of jazz, for example, that it should be worth hearing, that it has elements of surprise, and that it breaks out of predictable patterns – a point that may shed light on what is different about impulsivity. Just as spontaneity is constitutive of jazz, it may be constitutive of freedom and the good life (e.g., Kant 1933). Impulsivity, to the extent that it leads to actions one 'can't help' but do, or that one finds very, very hard to resist, hampers agency and autonomy, values central to freedom and the good life by most accounts.

Brown seems to distinguish between spontaneity and impulsivity, as when he discusses Glen Gould's antipathy toward live performances and explains that Gould was probably worrying about 'how one of his live performances could be deformed by impulsively plunging in at too fast a pace to suit the subsequent phrasing he thought the work required' (Brown 1996, p. 363).

Brown's point was that Gould was worried because of the mode of music he was committed to; jazz musicians take risks that, in fact, may take a suddenly bad turn, as when Louis Armstrong 'rushes too quickly, if thrillingly, into the first notes of the introduction in his famous Okeh recording of *West End Blues*' (1996, p. 365). With spontaneity, risky behavior can turn out badly too. So what is different?

Brown argues that a key aspect of creating jazz is the musician's self-monitoring in the midst of the creative act: 'With improvisational perform-ance, one's concern is about how a player's on-the-spot decisions and actions create the very music unfolding as one listens' (1996, p. 364).

The idea that, even in the throes of spontaneous improvisation, the jazz musician is monitoring the creative moment in the context of a larger meaning may be related to the earlier discussion of everyday ordinary actions as situated within a life plan or long-term goals. Although I resist the overly rational pic-ture of deliberation and action as always situated within larger plans and aims, I think there is something important in the self-monitoring that Brown talks about that may be lacking or weak in impulsively acting people. I here intro-duce the Olaf principle as a possible way to mark the difference between impul-sivity and spontaneity. This idea is most closely related to Neely's ideas of higher order desires where desires are prioritized.

The Olaf principle was coined by Lynne McFall (1987), after an e.e. cum-mings poem. Olaf, in this poem, is a conscientious objector who refuses to fight in a war and is tortured by the military for being a coward. Here is the relevant part:

> Olaf (upon what were once knees)
> Does almost ceaselessly repeat
> 'there is some s. I will not eat'
>
> (Cummings 1926, p. 37)

The idea is that some of the commitments we hold are more important to us than are others. Those commitments that we hold dear but can be sacrificed without remorse McFall calls defeasible commitments; Sally loves her profes-sional life and is deeply committed to it, but if her partner needed her to be home to take care of him, she would do so. On the other hand, McFall says, 'there are things we could not do without self-betrayal and personal disinte-gration' (1987, p. 13). She calls these 'identity-conferring' commitments. The idea that some of our commitments are defeasible and some are not is helpful in thinking through impulsivity and spontaneity in the context of overall well-being. For what seems to be the primary difference is that, with spontaneous behavior, one preserves the desire for overall well-being (as in the jazz musician whose improvisations are self-monitored such that norms for jazz are maintained). Impulsivity may clash with the Olaf principle because even though one makes commitments not to do certain kinds of things, like engage in self-injurious behavior, those commitments turn out to be defeasible. An impulsive person may not be able to keep unconditional commitments due to impulses. To the extent that violating the Olaf principle erodes one's sense of self, it feeds distress. What makes impulsivity undesirable, then, is not based on an outcome, but on the threat it poses to our ability to hold onto a sense of identity. We might find that the Olaf principle, coupled with impulsivity, may correlate with the BPD criterion of identity disturbance. On the other hand, if we conceptualize impulsivity as holding commitments that one then violates, we may be mapping it onto the moral domain as lack of integrity or untrustworthiness, moving us away from an understanding of impulsivity as a mental disorder.

4.7 Impulsivity, gender, and sexuality

In this section, I bring in research on gender and sexuality as a way to understand how complex is the issue of impulsivity when evaluating BPD women's behavior. Examining sexual behaviors is just one way to unpack impulsivity; earlier in this chapter I have used the examples of Rachel's running out barefoot at night and Maggie's cutting herself after deciding not to cut. The two forms of sexual behavior I consider are multiple sex partners (aka promiscuity) and casual sex (sex without strings).

I propose to enlist a discussion of transgression and conformity in an analysis of BPD impulsivity. The idea is that BPD patients are 75% female. One characteristic of these patients is impulsivity. One form that impulsivity takes, it is thought, is promiscuous sex and casual sex. Impulsive casual sex is more likely to also be unsafe sex due to lack of planning – but we've already seen that impulsive behavior doesn't necessarily involve lack of planning. It seems to have more to do with desires one cannot override, or has an extremely difficult time overriding – the 'irresistible desires' idea – or having flawed belief systems about some kinds of actions. Is it helpful to think of women who engage in casual, perhaps risky, sex as acting on irresistible desires or as having flawed belief systems about certain kinds of actions? Maybe impulsive casual sex that women engage in means they are nymphomaniacs, to use an outdated term, or are hypersexual, as they are now called (Rinehart 1997). Or maybe the story is more complicated than that.

I begin by returning to a discussion of cultural norms, this time, in terms of representations of sexuality and how they intersect with gender. Media including television, movies, music, magazines and, now, the Internet provide the primary sex education for adolescents, where sex is depicted as frequent, glamorous, and free of consequences (Brown *et al.* 2006). And, because these messages remain fairly constant, those who spend a good portion of their days using these media may come to believe that those norms reflect the actual world and to adopt those norms as their own; this result is more the case for white teens than for black ones, as black youth seem more responsive to parental and religious attitudes and norms (Brown *et al.* 2006, p. 1025).

A widespread result of media depictions of sex and sexuality is that casual sex is on the rise: large numbers of youth have their first sexual experience with someone they do not consider to be romantically involved with, and 70% of college students report having sexual intercourse with 'a friend' or someone they had 'just met' (Grello *et al.* 2006). Many describe such occasions as spontaneous or impulsive (interchangeably using those terms). Women, as well as men, engage in casual sex, but for different reasons and with different results on their well-being. Studies show that emotional investment is far more important for females than for males, so some researchers suggest that females may have casual sex in the hope of the relationship becoming closer and deeper as a result. Grello *et al.* (2006), for example, found that 52% of males compared to 36% of females in their study reported having casual sex, but females significantly differed in what they expected the outcome would be: 18% of females but only 3% of males thought that this casual sexual encounter was the beginning of a romance. On the other hand, over half of all males and females thought the casual sex was 'just a one-time thing.'

Girls considered intimacy significantly more important and sexual pleasure less significantly important than did boys. 'Young adolescents viewed intimacy, sexual pleasure and social status as important goals in a relationship, and many had strong expectations that sex would satisfy these goals. These goals and expectations differed by gender and sexual experience' (Ott *et al.* 2006, p. 87). That study, on what sorts of positive things adolescents expect to come from sex, and what they hope would follow from it, found clear evidence of a double standard (Ott *et al.* 2006, p. 87). Nevertheless, those researchers did find that young men also desire intimacy more than sexual pleasure – but not to the degree that young women do.

We know that, in most societies, what is considered sexual prowess and normal sex drive for males is considered promiscuous for females (cf. Walsh 1991; Hynie *et al.* 1998; and Impett and Peplau 2003). Christian Klesse analyzed what he refers to as 'anti-promiscuity discourse' and found that the discourse functions as a way for male-dominated societies to police female sexuality. 'Accusing a person of being promiscuous is part and parcel of a highly gendered, classed and racialized discourse on sexuality' (Klesse 2005, p. 449). Women who engage in casual sex and/or have multiple sexual partners are called sluts, slags, and whores, labels that signify impurity, unchastity, and dishonor (Klesse 2005). And in many parts of the world, sexually active women are considered unsuitable for marriage, a very undesirable outcome in cultures where women need economic support from men and where the only way to attain that support is through marriage.

Feona Attwood (2006) illustrates numerous ways in which contemporary North American and European societies are trying to shift the terms of sexualities. She argues that we cannot afford not to update the moral norms in our increasingly sexualized cultures. Sexualized culture is defined as:

> A contemporary preoccupation with sexual values, practices and identities; the public shift to more permissive sexual attitudes; the proliferation of sexual texts; the emergence of new forms of sexual experience; the apparent breakdown of rules, categories and regulations designed to keep the obscene at bay; our fondness for scandals, controversies, and panics around sex ....

(Attwood 2006, pp. 78–79)

But even though these cultures are increasingly sexualized, they retain a significant double standard for women.

Louisa Allen (2003) studied young adults to see the extent to which they accommodated societal expectations and norms for sexual behavior ('girls want love, boys want sex') and, alternatively, the extent to which they resist being 'normal' by society's standards. Her literature review calls attention to the persistent stereotypes of the undesiring woman and the virile but detached man. Some of her subjects position women as 'reluctant recipients of male desires' (2003, p. 220), while others rejected the equation of female sexual activity with sluttiness. Some young men joked about stereotypes of young male sexuality (always ready, always able), while others said that the thing they most want out of a (hetero) sexual relationship is love (2003, p. 228). But overall, significantly more women than men reported wanting caring, support, understanding, trust, honesty, and respect (2003, p. 230). Allen concludes that young people's sexual selves do not always conform to a sexual double standard, even though the double standard and sexual stereotypes are widely shared and enacted.

The worry is that norms and values about what female sexuality should and should not be may be leaking into judgments of impulsivity. It's not that an association between impulsive behavior and female casual sex cannot be found. It's that, unlike taking off on a run at night, our sexual behaviors are gender coded through and through. A woman who cannot modulate her sexual impulses [sic] may not be considered mentally ill but morally reprobate. On the other hand, we have seen a case in the United States of 23-year-old Debra Lafave, a middle-school teacher who had sex with a 14-year-old boy; her defense attorney, John Fitzgibbons, reasoned the following: 'Here we have a woman that, by every societal standard, can get a date. Can get a man. Yet, she destroyed her career, destroyed her marriage. I believe the only logical reason why Deborah Lafave did what she did was because of her mental illness.' [from Dateline NBC June 3, 2008] Cultures do not look favorably on either men or women who have sex with underage young people. But when it comes to women's sexual behavior, whether casual sex or with multiple sex partners, an explanation is called for. And the available options seem to be either that her sexual behavior is a symptom of a mental disorder or that it is a sign of moral weakness: she is a slut, a slag, and a whore – character terms.

4.8 Conclusion

Drawing on philosophical arguments, I have clarified what impulsive behavior is so that it can be better understood in clinical contexts. We can understand it as unvoluntary action due to an irrational but intractable belief or a gap between belief and motivation; or an inability to act on higher order desires due to irresistible desires; or to act on desires that are very, very hard to resist but are minimally resistable. Impulsivity doesn't necessarily mean 'unplanned.' Rachel and Maggie are impulsive, but Rachel is more so. Although impulsive behavior may involve risk-taking, it needn't do so. Furthermore, spontaneous behavior is also risky. It is also unplanned, but occurs within the context of self-monitoring for the limits of the domain. I introduced the Olaf principle, which is that some of our commitments are indefeasible, identity-conferring commitments. The Olaf principle might explain a difference between spontaneity and impulsivity in that the latter is an overriding of one's unconditional commitments. The worry here, though, is that this way of understanding impulsivity raises the 'mad or bad' problem discussed in the *Introduction*. To remind readers, this problem is one of determining when a psychiatric judgment of pathology has identified a genuine psychiatric condition and when, instead, such judgment contains moral values of social or cultural disapproval.[5] The issue, as John Sadler sets it out, is what degree of social deviance or unconventionality is enough to count as a mental disorder (cf. Sadler 2005, Ch. 6). An example from psychiatry is whether to include behavior such as pedophilia as a psychiatric condition or just a criminal one. In thinking about one impulsive BPD behavior, casual sex, we see this problem more clearly. Norms for

---

[5] ...or both, as Zachar and I argue (2009 forthcoming).

femaleness lead us to judge women who engage in casual sex much more harshly than we do men. Casual sex is not necessarily impulsive. But, because of those gendered norms for sexuality, when we find women who engage in casual sex or sex with multiple partners, we look for an explanation. Are they sluts (morally bad) or can't they help themselves (impulsive and mentally ill)? Or are they deliberatively and deliberately violating norms for gendered sexuality that they see as confining and oppressive?

Again drawing on the Olaf principle, I suggest that one thing that might help in distinguishing female casual sex as impulsive versus spontaneous would be to know whether or not the person holds an Olaf principle about casual sex. This principle might be something like, 'I will only have sex with someone after I've gotten to feel affection and closeness with him or her,' or 'I will only pick up people to have sex with once a year.' If they do hold such a principle and then they violate it, we might conclude that their behavior is impulsive. Here the connection between spontaneity and the Olaf principle is clear: behaviors are chosen – sometimes sudden and unexpected ones – within the context of self-monitoring and attention to a broader landscape of aims and directions. This may be applicable whether we are talking about jazz or sexual behavior.[6] However, if women who have casual sex don't hold an Olaf principle about it, it is an open question whether or not they are doing so impulsively. Clinicians should take into account the gendered sexual norms that set up an expectation that women who say they 'just can't resist' casual sex must have something wrong with them – cultural norms don't indicate this about men. Maybe women just really like sex and like it to be spontaneous. Are they exempt from being judged as morally bad? Maybe not, but that isn't in the domain of psychiatry.

As we have seen, sexual activity is only one way that BPD patients may be either impulsive, thereby exhibiting symptomatic behavior, or more deliberately transgressive, expressing defiance of cultural norms. Rachel is impulsive by taking off on her run, and what makes her behavior impulsive rather than spontaneous is that she doesn't seem to be engaging in any self-monitoring as to how this particular move will affect a larger picture nor does she seem either to consider her late night run an aspect of a defeasible commitment or a considered and chosen violation of an unconditional commitment. Maggie's cutting is more complicated; if we use the framework of the defeasible and unconditional commitments, Maggie might be seen as struggling with defeasible commitments

---

[6] A link between jazz and sexuality is sometimes made, including the assertion that the word 'jazz' originated as an expression for sexual intercourse. Nevertheless, the etymology of 'jazz' is unknown. See Merriam and Garner (1968) for a fascinating history of this word.

rather than with irresistible desires, where the therapeutic aim might be to shift a defeasible commitment not to cut to an unconditional commitment not to self-injure any more. Whether or not Maggie can be said to be struggling with competing commitments or with competing desires may depend, at least in part, with the degree to which Maggie considers her options for action within the context of a larger life plan. Or consider someone who becomes hostile and aggressive in the face of opposition to her expectations or aims, or (a messier problem) someone who is in substance abuse treatment and picks up that drink anyway. A person with such behavior must be considered not only in the light of a clearer understanding of what impulsivity is but also in light of that person's life context, aims, and defeasible and unconditional commitments if she holds them. My working theory of impulsivity, therefore, will need to be particularized to given patients, and then the theory modified in the light of grounded and everyday therapeutic experience.

Chapter 5

Self-injurious behavior

5.1 **The scope of the problem**

One of the more troubling activities that characterize people diagnosed with borderline personality disorder is self-injury. Self-injurious behaviors (SIB) also show up in some other personality disorders (Favazza 1989) and psychiatric conditions (Favazza 1996), but this analysis focuses on the intersection between BPD and self-injury. As John Gunderson says, the criterion of self-mutilating behavior 'is so prototypical of persons with BPD that the diagnosis rightly comes to mind whenever recurrent self-destructive behaviors are encountered' (2001, p. 11). In order to know how to respond to people who are self-injurious, clinicians need to know what it is. And it's trickier to answer that question than one might think. Many definitions of actions falling in this category tend to be question-begging, as this chapter will suggest. Alderman (1997) summarizes self-injurious behavior as acts that are done to oneself, performed by oneself, physically violent, not suicidal, and intentional and purposeful. But that definition includes too much, such as culturally sanctioned practices (cf. Favazza 1996). The literature distinguishes between 'delicate' or superficial and severe self-mutilation, which is defined as 'the deliberate infliction of direct physical injury on one's own body...that involves cutting, maiming, destroying or altering a part of one's body in a socially unacceptable fashion, and [which] may result in permanent disfigurement' (Parrott and Murray 2001, p. 317). One of the things that needs to be disentangled is the role that the designation of 'socially unacceptable' behavior plays in marking a difference between kinds of body modification. If self-injurious behavior cannot be understood independent of the rubric of socially unacceptable behavior, it is a question-begging concept. But, as Armondo Favazza states, 'Self-mutilation has been trivialized (wrist-cutting), regarded merely as a symptom (borderline personality disorder), and misreported by the media and the public' (Favazza 1998, p. xii). So, in taking up the question of what marks off socially acceptable and unacceptable body modification, I must take care not to make those mistakes.

Causes of self-injury are unclear. The most commonly supported explanatory theories are that such acts are kinds of ritual, symbolic expressions, or tension relieving (Zila and Kiselica 2001). Ross and McKay (1979) offer an array of possible causes of self-mutilation including ritual and symbolism, sex, regression, existential statement, manipulation, risk taking, attention seeking, retaliation, frustration, depression, tension relief, inappropriate communication, self-punishment, and low self-esteem (listed in Zila and Kiselica 2001). I would also think that impulsive behavior should be on this list. Diana Milia places self-injury in the 'context of cycles of creation and destruction inherent within the creative process' and argues that its healing potential arises out of transformative elements that parallel ritual and other creative processes (2000, p. 12). Another theory posits self-injuring acts as an externalization of a woman's fears of being a passive victim of bodily attacks. On this view, fears grounded in a female physiology that is experienced as unruly and particularly vulnerable to invasion are defended against by being the one in control of the harm (Cross 1993). In general, the better attempts to understand cutting and other self-injuring activities view self-injury as employing a form of 'default' rationality. On this view, what the person does is rational given her history and the way she views the world, but she acts in ways that are not consistent with norms for living a flourishing life. As a response to trauma, cutting and other forms of self-injuring are highly adaptive responses. For example, Janice McLane (1996) argues that self-mutilation allows a trauma victim a 'voice on the skin' when she is otherwise feeling silenced. On this view, the cutting 'says' what the woman cannot put into words. The body, then, is being used to communicate something that is difficult or impossible to articulate in conventional modes (Crowe and Bunclark 2000; Milia 2000, p. 76; Miller 1994).

I suggest a way of thinking about self-injury that takes seriously its potentially destructive aspects while situating it in a broader discourse of body modifications where the body is being used as a text. Favazza (1996) has already provided an extended and thorough analysis of body modifications within cultural contexts, so I try not to duplicate his efforts. Instead, this chapter focuses on the question of what it means to say that body modifications are a kind of communication and why we should think that some ways we communicate are 'better' than others.

To say that the body is a text is to suggest that the body, like other mediums of communication, must be interpreted and that its meanings are not given or inevitable. 'As a field of interpretive possibilities, the body is a locus of the dialectical process of interpreting anew a historical set of interpretations which have already informed corporeal style. The body becomes a peculiar nexus of culture and choice, and "existing" one's body becomes a personal way of taking up and reinterpreting received gender norms' (Butler 1987, pp. 133–134; see also Bordo 1989). On this view, one of the texts by which we communicate and engage in mutual meaning-making is the body. This way of framing self-injury raises questions about the role popular culture and psychiatry play in imbuing some acts as fashionable, others as transgressive, and still others as pathological. It also brings into focus the increasing treatment of the body as a commodity and complex attitudes people have about bodies. My aim is to open up a space for clinicians to be able to respond to a patient who is self-injuring in a morally grounded and therapeutically effective way, drawing upon explanatory theories like the above to some extent but not letting them stand in for the hard work of interactive patient/clinician communication. Treatment is unlikely to be both ethical and effective until more attention is paid to these patients' own views of their behavior (Miller 1994). The task for clinicians – both a therapeutic and moral one – is to find out what, if anything, the *patient* means by the signs with which she communicates. Readers were introduced to the concept of uptake in Chapter 2, and it is a relevant concept here, too. Behavior that seems to be self-injurious requires that clinicians give uptake to what the patient says she means by her behavior. In Part II of the book, I flesh out the idea of giving uptake as a virtue that clinicians will find useful in working with BPD patients.

5.2 Meaning-making and responsibility: Part one

It is widely recognized that how we experience the world is shaped by our conceptual scheme. This observation has led some philosophers as well as some clinicians to take the further step of claiming that what we believe is true – what we count as knowledge – is (at least partly) determined by our conceptual scheme. On this view, in forming our beliefs – what we take to be true – we are not just passively impinged upon by an independently structured world but instead, through our conceptual scheme, we in some sense *construct* our representations of reality. The idea is that knowledge is not determined by the nature of things (Hacking 1999, p. 6); or that what we count as knowledge is always, to some degree, mediated by the particularity of knowers (Code 1991); or that any division between natural kinds and social production of those kinds is *a priori* indefensible (Gillett 1999, p. 73). It is important to note that a claim that knowledge is socially mediated does not commit one to relativism: still there are ways to get things right or wrong (such as that sexism and racism exist in social institutions and profoundly shape our lives; cf. Code 1991). It does, however, lead to the idea that how we interpret things is not independent of the social milieu in which beliefs, ideas, and values emerge, and that what we perceive, when we interact in the world, is always already mediated by norms and practices. Many clinicians are keenly aware that their perceptions, interpretations, and responses to patients are shaped by larger social and cultural contexts as well as value-laden theories of health and rationality. But it may be difficult to see how ideas about social epistemology can be applied to people who engage in self-injury. I believe that the framework is illuminating in that it allows us to reorient a discussion of ethical responses to such cases. The connection, as I see it, is that the relationship between communicating and knowing requires that we be epistemically responsible, not just morally responsible. I make a case for this in Chapter 7.

5.2.1 Communicating with/on/by the body

First, let me say something about body communications since that is the domain of inquiry. Traditional philosophical analyses of communication focused primarily on speech acts and paid little or no attention to nonlinguistic signs. Critics, however, have argued that this way of conceptualizing communication is too narrow and that we employ numerous other modes of communicative interaction. We communicate through styles of dress, for example, through body 'language,' smoke signals, and with gift-giving. Each of the various modes of communication raises ethical questions about norms for communicating with one another. In order to foster respect, friendliness, and community, communicative ethics must make a place for 'gestures that bring people together warmly, seeing conditions for amicability: smiles, handshakes, hugs, the giving and taking of food and drink' and other embodied nonlinguistic acts (Young 1996, p. 129). But it is important not to take the norms at the face value: they vary from culture to culture, are gendered, and may carry biases and unwarranted assumptions. Clinicians are trained to pay attention to a variety of modes of communication and so are well positioned to apply a communicative ethics where the body plays a positive role. This chapter probes the norms for communication and accompanying assumptions with the aim of clarifying the role clinicians can play in addressing BPD patients' self-injurious behavior.

5.3 Signs and culture

To provide a framework for understanding people diagnosed with BPD who self-injure, I draw on a concept from theories of meaning: signification. Signification is a process through which we communicate; through the patterns and forms of signification, we deploy discourses – systems of thought and fields of cultural life that organize and produce our practices, hierarchies, and categories. Discursive formations are related to power. As Michel Foucault (1972) argues, discourse unfolds as rules of exclusion, rules that determine what can be said and not said, who has the right to speak on a given subject, what will constitute reasonable and what foolish actions, what will count as 'true' and what as false. So it is important for us to understand how women's experiences in society might give rise to using the body as a text (for example, to say what cannot be said in conventional ways) and how the field of psychiatry produces a particular understanding of self-injury that might close off some interpretations.

Signs comprise a signifier (marks on a page or sounds or movements) and a signified (what those marks or sounds or movements mean). The signified, then, is the sense or meaning inscribed in a term or gesture. The task of a potential listener is to determine whether or not something is being communicated and, if so, to interpret it. The listener or audience doesn't do this alone. He relies on linguistic and other conventions to infer meaning. Part of this reliance involves the assumption that the communicator is employing a particular sign because she believes her audience will recognize the intention to communicate and pair it up with the intended meaning. (For example, if I am lost and build three fires in a row, I am doing this because I think that someone seeing them will conclude that I want someone to recognize that sign and infer that I need help). But as W.V.O Quine (1960) argues, conventions do not just spring into being; they are brought into being by the behavior of the parties to a given convention. This means, on Quine's view, that 'facts' about behavior are not enough to determine whether a given understanding of that behavior is correct. Consequently, we can conclude that interpretation is required, and interpretation is not a science but, instead, an art. I like the way Grant Gillett characterizes the discursive view of communication, in which he says:

> ...locates a person in relation to a sphere of discourse and allows one to identify the position he or she is taking and the subjective relationships holding between the person and the context. These reveal how it is to be that person and what choices for perception and action present themselves in a given situation. This in turn illuminates relationships of power, reveals the content of any significations used to organize behaviour, and renders understandable the activity of the person concerned; it is as if one were to successfully locate a person on a map so that you and they both remarked, 'Ah, now I see where I am!'

> (Gillett 1999, pp. 28–29)

What I think is right about this way of understanding explanation (e.g., a patient's explanation of her self-injuring behavior) is that it situates the communicator and audience in a discursive field in a context of power relations. Yet the greater weight of explanatory power in interpretation and meaning-making should be placed in the hands of the person whose behavior calls for explanation. I'll return to these points later.

The body is one kind of text, and the things it does are units of meaning within a discursive field. With my body, I express the idea 'I am a woman' through a myriad of signs of femininity that others know how to read. Movements like soft, gentle hand gestures, touching the hair on one's head, crossing one's legs, and tilting one's head are conventional signs of femininity (cf. Butler 1990).

But we make mistakes in our interpretations of signs all the time, including mistakes about gender. Signifiers for gender are like signifiers for Santa Claus – although sense-making, neither refers to anything real. In fact, signification necessarily relies on the construction of a metaphysics that disguises the arbitrariness of its own processes (see Derrida 1981, pp. 30–32; 1974, 12–14). That is, signs get their meaning from their relation to other signs. We rely on conventions of meaning in order to communicate with one another, but we are too often seduced into thinking that those conventions are reliable. As Gillett says, 'it is clear that the realm of discourse is not only an interpersonal realm but also that it cannot be understood without paying some attention to its social and cultural context' (Gillett 1999, p. 31). For example, as I discussed in Chapter 2, Marilyn Frye argues that, because linguistic and cultural conventions equate women's anger with cuteness, over-emotionality, inappropriateness, or irrelevance, (or, we might add, bitchiness or hormonal changes), women's anger at moral injustices done to them do not get taken seriously and respectfully; instead, cultural norms allow men to minimize, trivialize, pathologize, mock, and ignore women's anger. When interpreting another's signs, then, we need to be skeptical about cultural imperatives to appeal to conventions that close off alternative meanings or that impose meaning in ways that rob the speaker of her voice.

In interpreting what I will call body signifiers, the first thing you need to ask is whether the signifier has any meaning. (That is, *is* it a sign?) If you determine that you are picking up a sign, your task is to interpret it. Even here, we can make mistakes. Consider an act of burping. In our culture, burps generally are not taken to be 'saying' anything. But cultural meanings of the burp vary, which suggests that even knowing when to take seriously a signifier is sometimes complex. We can also err by assuming that a signifier has meaning when it may not. Contrast my friend's utterance 'one strawberry ice-cream, please' with the signifier 'butterfly tattoo' on her left breast. I might ask why she ordered strawberry ice cream as opposed to, say, chocolate, but her answer is likely to satisfy me without my needing to probe for more: she just likes it; it is a matter of taste. The tattoo might be a bit more difficult for me to appreciate; the answer 'Tattoos look cool' is a matter of opinion that I may find harder to wrap my mind around. But if I were to push her on the meaning of tattooing in her life, I seem to be assuming that tattooing is not like eating ice cream – a matter of taste – but that it signifies something that requires further explanation. When I decide that signifying 'coolness' isn't enough of an answer, I may be looking for deeper meaning that just isn't there. But as I've said, we don't make decisions in a cultural vacuum about whether, in a given situation, to accept the relativity of taste or, rather, to press for further explanations: cultural norms influence our interpretations and responses to others' signifying acts.

5.4 When is self-injury an act of communication? What is it communicating?

The going wisdom about self-injury is that the person engaging in such acts *is* trying to say something. My first point, then, is that this general assumption should not be made universal. Research suggests that some self-injury may be merely a response to physiological stimuli, so not all self-injury has meaning. But secondly, interpretations of self-injurious acts tend to appeal to a restricted domain of meaning that assumes an underlying psychological anguish in the actor. Although difficult for me to imagine, I believe it is logically possible for someone to enjoy the experience of watching blood drops form on her arm after cutting herself–and for her cutting to hold no other meaning than an aesthetic one. In fact, Favazza (1996) cites a report by Kafka of a young woman who felt herself to become 'sharply alive' at the moment of cutting herself:

> She described the flow of blood as being like a voluptuous bath whose pleasant warmth spread over her body, molding its contour and sculpting its form. She was at a loss to understand why everyone did not indulge in blood baths, especially since they were readily accessible simply by "unzipping" one's skin.

(Favazza 1996, p. 161)

But meaning-making is cultural and communal, and an assertion that one's self-injurious act is merely aesthetic may not be enough for others to let the matter rest. We draw on values and beliefs when interpreting signs, but what warrant do we have for aligning a given value or belief with a particular signifier? As Favazza says:

> our perceptions of self-mutilation are often unconsciously linked not only with the fear, revenge, mob violence, and governmental power associated with mutilation in general but also with concepts such as sacredness, self-knowledge, and the power of blood to heal and to bind individuals together.

(Favazza 1996, p. 4)

When we interpret signs written on the body, we must be skeptics with respect to cultural and linguistic norms. When a person is expressing something by cutting or burning herself, we need to remain open to what she may – and may not – be saying. We need critically to attend to the conventions we draw upon to interpret such signs and to question the cultural norms that delineate when it is and is not acceptable for a person to injure herself with the goal of giving herself aesthetic pleasure.

In the next section, I illustrate how complex the matter of the body as a text can be.

5.5 Situating self-injury

The deployment of the body as a text is not unique to those with personality disorders. Body modifications can represent aesthetic, religious, or political values. These days, people tattoo themselves, get body piercing and penile enhancement, color their hair purple, lighten (or darken) their skin, and go on starvation diets. Historically, religious people have fasted, flagellated themselves, and 'discovered' stigmata as signs of deep conviction. Lakota people have practiced sundance rituals. Protesters and laborers have gone on hunger strikes. In all these cases, the body is being used as a text. And in all cases, some degree of risk-taking and pain are involved. But interpreting the various signs is messy and complicated indeed. Is tattooing, for example, a fashionable form of self-expression or a sign of pathology (Sanders 1989; Inch and Huws 1993).

Let's consider an array of intentional actions that bring about body modifications, all of which involve some degree of risk and pain.

1. Tattooing
2. Body piercing
3. Surgical implants
4. Scarification
5. Pigmentation changes (skin lightening or tanning)
6. Radical dieting
7. Hunger striking
8. Fasting
9. Stigmata inducing
10. Cutting and burning[1]

Several points emerge from this list of kinds of body modifications. In each kind, in order to understand what is being 'said,' we have to consider not only the cultural norms that shape meaning and interpretation but also the individual speaker. What is being said and how it is meant to be received cannot be

---

[1] Some of these body modifications may be considered ornamental (body piercing in the United States; scarification in some African cultures), and some of these body modifications serve to identify group memberships (scarification may signify a particular ethnic identity; tattooing may signify belonging to a self-chosen community).

easily identified. For example, there are theories about the cultural meanings of tattooing and of scarification, but they offer hypotheses of general public meanings that may not be applicable to given individuals. A person with a tattoo may not be clear what her intentions are with regard to the tattoo, or she may not be intending to produce any effects on others. Many kinds of body modifications are imitative, and although meanings are constructed (often *post hoc*), a participant may not intend to say anything other than a reflexive 'me too.' Note, too, that the question 'Why did you do such-and-such an act of self-injury?' can be answered in terms either of explanation/motive or of meaning/intention to communicate, and this ambiguity creates its own problems in interpretation. If I offer an explanation in response to your 'why,' but you continue to seek for a deeper meaning, which of us should decide when the question has been answered? When ought an answer be sufficient to satisfy others?

I also observe that these actions can be grouped in various ways.

(a) The first five as 'amateur or professional' whereas the last five as 'self-injuring.'

(b) The first six as 'aesthetic,' the next one 'political,' the next two 'religious,' and the last one 'pathological.'

(c) The sixth and the tenth as 'pathological' and the rest as 'socially acceptable.'

Furthermore, some kinds of body modifications don't lend themselves to any of the above groupings in an obvious way. Amputation for non-medical reasons seems to be sought for reasons of identity rather than purely aesthetic or other reasons. For example, one person says 'My left foot was not part of me' to explain the desire for amputation (cf. Elliott 2000). Penile enhancement may also be sought as a matter of identity or self-worth. Are body modifications that are identity-affirming still self-injuring? Why would one kind (penile enhancement) be socially acceptable while the other (amputation) be pathological? Complicating these groupings even more is the claim by some tattooed people that their tattoos are an expression of identity (Bell 1999; Sanders 1989). Do these different identity-conferring 'self-injurious acts' have something in common that we do not understand?

It's not clear what justifies these groupings. Clearly, attitudes about what is proper and acceptable to do with one's body play an important role in interpretations of body signs. In tattooing, for example, even if the signified is about belonging, the tattoo is part of how its signification gets interpreted. We signify belonging in many ways: T-shirts, bumper stickers, and flags, for instance. When the signifier is written on the body, its materiality is itself important.

The chosen mode of signification, therefore, is part of the signified. Yet it's not clear what criteria we use in assigning sense and meaning to these various body signs.

As a culture, audience responses to this variety of body modifications are sometimes tolerant, other times oddly intractable. If we view a body alteration as aesthetic, political, religious, or identity-conferring, we may negatively evaluate it but eventually seem to drum up toleration. In those cases (students with nipple piercings, colleagues who fast), we make an effort to be tolerant even when we don't ourselves appreciate or understand or endorse the sign. This is even true of the excessively thin models, who evoke admiration and envy (but not judgments of pathology) in virtually everyone but health experts. What is so objectionable about cutting or burning that it cannot elicit tolerance like (for instance) scarification of some African cultures?

Let me give a preliminary answer to that question by way of two examples.

(1) Helen Miller was a 29-year-old woman released from incarceration and soon after was sentenced again, this time for grand larceny. She wanted to be placed in an asylum, so she began cutting herself. Armando Favazza reports that

> at final count ninety-four pieces of glass, thirty-four splinters, four shoe nails, one pin, and one needle had been removed from her arms....She felt no pain when inflicting her wounds and seemed to experience erotic pleasure whenever the doctors were forced to probe her flesh to remove objects.
>
> (Favazza 1996, p. 158)

> (2) An 18-year-old youth with no previous psychiatric history was found wandering in the street nude with his right eyeball in his hand. He had taken LSD for four consecutive days, during which he was forced into a homosexual episode. He then felt that he was going to die, that the devil controlled his mind, and that he should obey the Bible and pluck out his eye because he had offended God.
>
> (Favazza 1996, p. 102)

I offer those two examples to give readers an idea of the seriousness of some self-injurious behavior. Self-enucleation, for whatever reason, is rightfully disturbing, in that it intentionally and permanently damages one of the senses we need to function. Causing permanent and irreversible tissue damage to one's body also seems perverse – but here the case is more complex: tattooing also causes permanent tissue damage, and although tattoos can be removed, the technique generally leaves scars. Sun dances also cause permanent and irreversible tissue damage but are not deemed pathological because their cultural meaning is celebratory. So, although the above examples highlight the severity of certain behaviors, they are not definitively symptomatic. We still need to situate self-injurious behavior within historical, religious, and cultural traditions.

Blood-letting has ancient communal roots that merit examination in this context. Zila and Kiselica note that ritual and symbolism is one of two most commonly supported theories about causes of self-injury (the other being tension relief). Those authors, drawing on earlier research, note that

> 'Ross and McKay (1979) explained ritual and symbolism in descriptions of self-mutilation that are laden with religious overtones and symbolism. Favazza and Conterio (1989) concurred with this theory, citing frequent references to the need to atone for sins by those who self-mutilate. Himber (1994) found a common theme of self-purification among these individuals'

(Zila and Kiselica 2001)

There are many reasons a community engages in blood sacrifice, including pacification of afflicted spirits (Turner 1967) or payment of homage, atonement, or purification to deities (Burkert 1983). I will discuss one theory of sacrifice that may illuminate some self-injurious behavior.

Milia argues that, although sacrifice and symbolism have recognized cultural currency, one purpose of sacrifice is to draw boundaries between good and bad violence and to re-establish order for a community. Sacrifice, then, is a special kind of violence that the community approves of and controls through ritual and symbolism (Milia 2000, p. 17). The need to create order out of chaos and thus reassure requires that violence and blood-letting be further designated as good or bad kinds:

> Just as violence has been split into good and bad types–that which is sanctioned for the purpose of maintaining societal order and that which is unlawful–blood has also been classified in opposite types...The dual nature of blood becomes apparent as its presence represents the life force, and its spillage heralds the draining away of life.

(Milia 2000, p. 18)

What is striking in Milia's account is the suggestion that the transformative quality of sacrifice and its symbolism is in its duality. 'Symbolically, the sacred victim [of sacrifice] comes to represent that which is both evil and transcendent of evil. The ritual of sacrifice forms a bridge to transcendence of sin, and in this way accomplishes purification' (2000, p. 17). This analysis, then, suggests that the sign may not be just one thing – it may contain paradoxical concepts – and clinicians will need to look for contradictory meanings (and not push for an artificial or early resolution).

Still, the question remains why body modifications are given the meanings they are. Milia suggests that, even when mainstream culture views some body modifications as socially deviant or transgressive, they aren't viewed as pathologies if they are meaningful at least to a subculture. Tattooing, scarification, and body piercing are signs that transform self-injuring wounds into aesthetic expressions. This transformation purifies its violence and re-enacts rituals of human sacrifice at a higher level of symbolism (Milia 2000, p. 26). Cutting or burning, however, and certainly self-enucleation, when done alone and in secret, fall outside culturally acceptable meanings of aesthetic, ritual, or political significance (Milia 2000, p. 43).

Furthermore, contemporary culture has generated panic and distrust about bodily fluids, displacing fears about external threats onto the secreting, leaky body.

> The *rubber gloves* the Washington police force insisted on wearing before touching the bodies of gays who were arrested at recent AIDS demonstrations in Lafayette Park across from Reagan's White House; the *sexual secretions* in contemporary American politics where presidential candidates, from Hart to Celeste, are condemned out of hand by a media witch hunt focusing on unauthorized sexual emissions; and *routine testing*, the Reagan Administration's bureaucratic term for the mandatory policing of the bodies of immigrants, prison populations, and members of the armed services who are to be put under (AIDS) surveillance for the slightest signs of the breakdown of their immunological systems.
>
> (Kroker 1987, 12; emphasis in original)

The distinction between 'good' and 'bad' body modifications, therefore, may indicate cultural responses to perceived evil or impending danger. Nevertheless, as Milia suggests, the distinction really seems to amount to a difference between what a culture understands and does not understand (or between what it is willing to understand or not).

Finally, while I am not arguing for a new taxonomy for BPD, I do think that this broader view of body modifications suggests that the term 'self-injury' (or 'self-mutilation' for that matter) doesn't pick out a persuasive set of factors for pathologizing body-related actions of someone diagnosed with BPD. I suggest that self-injurious behavior in BPD patients should be investigated for its potential association with impulsivity as I defined it in Chapter 4. Two problems arise then: first, someone whose body is covered with tattoos could also be viewed as exhibiting SIB (she 'can't help' but get another tattoo), and then it seems we're back to the problem of conflating culture with pathology that I raised in previous chapters and second, we know that neither impulsivity nor SIB is unique to BPD. These problems make it difficult to know what factors are being validly correlated when doing research.

Historically and cross-culturally, then, there is a variety of potentially harmful body modifications, and they intersect with cultural norms in complex and varied ways. The next section situates self-injury more broadly in the context of cultural, political, and economic attitudes about the body.

5.6 **Commodity/body/sign**

In this section, I consider the possibility that some self-injurious actions have meaning but argue that that meaning may indicate cultural, rather than individual, pathologies. Where body modifications are concerned (cutting and burning included), self-injuring may signify a reaction against dehumanization (Milia 2000, p. 47). One theory of self-injuring suggests that, by harming the body, the individual highlights a distinction between body and self (Zila and Kiselica 2001).

The typical self-injurer is female, adolescent or young adult, single, from a middle to upper-middle class family, and intelligent (Suyemoto and MacDonald 1995; Favazza and Conterio 1989). One study found that the difference between BPD patients who engaged in self-mutilation and those who did not could not be explained by different histories of abuse or by levels of dissociation (Zweig-Frank et al. 1994). Rather than looking for meanings that go back to childhood experiences, clinicians might explore ways that the culture produces what is viewed as self-injurious behavior. Like tattooing and other accepted forms of body modification, cutting and burning may be imitated actions and, in fact, research suggests that social contagion may be a factor in self-injury (Favazza 1996; Zweig-Frank et al. 1994). But instead of signifying a contagion of individual pathological behavior, it may signify those individuals' locations in social and economic systems. Because most of BPD patients who self-injure are female, I focus here on female bodies.

Robert Mitlitsch (1998) argues that late capitalism has amplified a commodification of the body. The sign-value of the body has increasingly come to hold aesthetic promise as well as the use/exchange value. Commodification, then, performs the cultural labor of signification. As the global economy becomes increasingly consumer oriented, and the body is conceptualized as another commodity to market and re-make as desirable, the body is susceptible to objectification as never before (for just one example, see Morgan 1991).

Women's bodies are commodified specifically in sexual ways. (Women's bodies are also commodified in the service of reproduction, but I don't go into that issue here). Women still internalize cultural views that their primary value is in evoking sexual desire and delivering up sexual pleasure. Normative femininity includes standards of beauty that position women of value as impossibly thin and attractive. Whether or not an individual woman resists these norms, she must objectify herself in order to evaluate herself and decide how to respond to those norms.

The distress expressed by women diagnosed with BPD may not be unique but rather may reflect a more general experience of being female in our culture (Miller 1994). The female body in the literature and popular culture has been both extolled and despised, eroticized and reified, and yet viewed with disgust and distrust. Female being is conceptualized and represented as a being-to-be-perceived (Bourdieu 2001; Bartky 1990; Kaplan 1983; Berger 1972). Body image, for many women, is fragmented into parts (a pretty waist, an ugly nose) rather than as a whole, embodied self (Cross 1993). This claim is borne out by research on attitudes self-injuring women have about their bodies: 'More than half of the [self-injuring] participants in Favazza and Conterio's (1989) study reported the presence of troublesome sexual feelings: 34% hated their breasts, 56% strongly hated having a pelvic exam, and 10% indicated they would be better off without a vagina' (Zila and Kiselica 2001). But these findings are not specific to those who self-injure. Body loathing is not surprising given cultural attitudes about women's bodies.

Furthermore, female physiology contributes to women's experiences of their bodies as discontinuous and alien. Partially internal genitalia, with their ambiguous and mysterious workings, relatively abrupt changes in body contours during puberty and pregnancy, and menstruation with its pain and messiness give rise to experiences of embodiment that are ambivalent at best. Female physiology intersects with a culture that, in particular, commodifies women's bodies, over-determining a metaphysics of the body as an object.

In the context of an economy and culture where body commodification and objectification proliferates, women become increasingly alienated from their bodies (see, for example, Emberley 1987). Hence, the need increases for women to experience their bodies as real. This can prompt a (perhaps unconscious) transgressive response in an attempt to realize the body as 'one's own.' ('Trangression' is used here in the cultural sense, rather than in the sense of sin and evil, and is sometimes used to praise acts that violate repressive norms. For a discussion on an ethos of transgressive acts as acts of resistance to socially controlled and disciplined bodies, see Passerin-d'Entreves 1999; see also Marchak 1990). Judith Butler, drawing on Mary Douglas's theory of the body, says that whenever boundaries of the body are established, the taboos about the limits of those bodies become naturalized (made to seem natural) (Butler 1990, p. 131). And Douglas, in a passage that resonates with Milia's analysis of the duality in sacrifice, writes that 'ideas about separating, purifying, demarcating and punishing transgressions have as their main function to impose system on an inherently untidy experience. It is only by exaggerating the difference between within and without, above and below, male and female, with and against, that a semblance of order is created' (Douglas, as quoted in

Butler 1990, p. 131). The point is that what constitutes the limit of the body is signified by taboos and anticipated transgressions (Butler 1990, p. 131).

Self-injury is a taboo because it transgresses an imposed boundary that seems, to us, natural and given – the boundary between body and self, between material and immaterial, and between subject and object. Favazza cites Winnicott, who understands a woman who ate pieces of her fingers as an 'experiencing' of an intermediate and ongoing aspect of life where we must both keep inner and outer reality separate and also know it as interrelated (Favazza 1996, p. 161). The problem of where boundaries of the self are and how to understand their fluidity that I first discussed in Chapter 1 exerts itself here again. And as the body is increasingly destabilized and disposable, it requires more and greater transgressive acts to produce the appearance of substance. Cutting and burning, then, might be understood as an attempt to 'own the body, to perceive it as self (not other), known (not uncharted and unpredictable), and impenetrable (not invaded or controlled from the outside)' (Cross 1993). Still, these interpretations may not be what an individual woman means when she cuts or burns; asked why she cuts herself, an individual may not explain things this way. And clinicians may still want to convince her not to resist commodification *this* way, arguing for better ways to produce the appearance of substance. My point is that the audience is unlikely to learn the meaning of the sign in a given situation unless it learns to listen differently – to give uptake to the patient's meaning-making.

5.7 Conclusion

Clinicians are often at a loss to understand the actions of individuals who self-injure. Many find that it is difficult to talk about self-injury in a way that allows the patient a role as interpreter of her own signs (Favazza 1996; Himber 1994). 'Ross and McKay (1979) found that only after conceding that they did not understand self-mutilation were counselors then able to suspend clinical judgment and allow the young women to explain their behavior' (Zila and Kiselica 2001). Being a good clinician involves not only therapeutic skill and ethical commitments, but also an adherence to good epistemic practices. To be epistemically responsible is to seek out knowledge, acknowledging the limitations of our individual and professional body of knowledge. It is to ask ourselves questions about who gets to count as knowers and to work toward egalitarian knowledge production and attitudes toward variously positioned knowers. It is to resist prevailing psychiatric discourse when its power to pathologize is uncalled for. I say more on this issue in Part II of the book. For now, I just emphasize the importance of clinicians' approaching patients with a degree of epistemic humility.

BPD patients, the population relevant to our examination, need much guidance in order to work through their many difficulties and suffering. But they also need to be encouraged to see themselves as would-be knowers. And to do this, they must be the ones to say what they mean to communicate (or not) about their behaviors that look like self-injury. This does not mean that whatever they say must be right (see 5.2 above), but that the discursive power that silences women in many ways must be shifted to the patients to some degree.

Chapter 6

What's wrong with being manipulative?

6.1 Introduction to the problem

Manipulativity is not a diagnostic criterion for borderline personality disorder. Nevertheless, it is ubiquitous in the literature when discussing and describing patients and this disorder. In fact, 'so frequently does the word crop up in conversations and discourse about such patients, that it might wrongly be thought of as the major problem that such patients pose to psychiatric services, or the major defining criteria of their disorder' (Bowers 2003, p. 323). Typical of the literature is the following description of the behavior of patients who are considered to have BPD. Their …

> … behavior was judged as unadaptive to the interview. They did things to hinder the interview, such as asking questions irrelevant to its purpose, getting up and changing chairs, or refusing to answer questions. They behaved in predominantly angry ways, expressing anger toward a variety of targets, including the interviewer. They were argumentative, irritable, and sarcastic. Without tact or consideration, they were demanding and attempted to manipulate the interviewer to acquiesce to their wishes.
>
> (Perry and Klerman 1980, p.168)

The described behaviors are at least different in degree, if not in kind, from self-injurious behavior or suicide threats, the *sine qua non* of BPD patients. Yet clinicians tend to equate BPD patients with manipulativity and to forewarn others about them. For example, one researcher claims to distinguish BPD patients from depressed or schizophrenic ones by 'their angry, demanding, and entitled presentation,' and another warns that 'any interviewer, whether with a clinical or research purpose, will be exposed to devaluation, manipulation, angry outbursts, clinging or appeal' (Mitton and Huxley 1988). Most bluntly, 'borderliners are the patients you think of as PIAs–pains in the ass' (*Medical World News* 1983). As I will show, what clinicians and staff mean by 'manipulative behavior' varies widely. Because manipulativity is a pejorative term and because it refers to behavior that is thought to require 'management,' the use of the term needs to be more precise. The aim of this chapter is to isolate the behavior most appropriately called manipulative and to identify reasons why it might be a problem for patients to be manipulative. Current clinical usage collapses the distinction between moral values about wrong behavior and clinical values about psychological dysfunction, and part of the task is analytically to separate those two domains.

6.2 **An example**

To open the enquiry, let's consider the following transcript. This exchange takes place the night before the first scheduled appointment between a therapist and a BPD patient because the patient experiences a medical emergency. Here is the exchange:

> Ms. A: You could be dying before you got any help around here! My arm is killing me! This place is crazy!
> Therapist: Ms. A, I would like to introduce myself. I am Dr. Wheelis.
> Ms. A: Oh, no kidding! I didn't expect you. You're a resident? Interesting. You must be either very good or very crazy to have taken me on.
> Therapist: I can't tell if that's an invitation, a warning, or both [patient smiled at the comment], but we have an appointment tomorrow. Why don't we discuss it then. For now, perhaps I should take a look at your arm.
> Ms. A: No, it's okay, just a little bang.
> Therapist: Are you sure? You suggested that it was giving you considerable pain.
> Ms. A: No, it's fine, really. I'll see you tomorrow. By the way, I hate being called Ms. A.
> Therapist: How would you like to be called?
> Ms. A: Lotta. That's what everyone calls me.
> Therapist: Very well, as you wish.

> (Wheelis and Gunderson 1998)

An echo of Perry and Klerman's assessment of 'borderlines' can be found in the discussion of the transcript provided by Lotta's therapist and the co-author:

> Already in this initial interaction with Lotta's therapist-to-be, harbingers of the therapeutic challenges are evident. Ms. A demonstrates a manipulative style that predates the first interaction by seeking help through the exaggeration of a minor physical complaint. There is also the hint that Ms. A may be taking pleasure in suggesting to the therapist-to-be that working with her will be more than a small challenge. Her final request, to be called Lotta [rather than Ms. A] betrays her desire to bypass professional formality by requesting an immediate familiarity.

> (Wheelis and Gunderson 1998)

The commentary suggests that the therapist may have given more weight to the diagnostic category in which Lotta is said to fit than to the *particular person Lotta*. In such an encounter, the therapist sees markers of BPD: manipulativity, efforts to control others, repudiation of socially accepted boundaries, and resistance to socially approved conduct. But is it correct to characterize Lotta's behavior in this encounter as manipulative? And is her behavior dysfunctional, or just irritating?

6.3 **Conceptual cloudiness**

We cannot answer the question of what is wrong with manipulativity until we know what it is. In this section, I start with examples of the way the term is used with an eye to showing how sloppy its application is. Then, I offer a cleaner definition but one that leaves crucial questions unanswered about the distinction between dysfunctional and morally objectionable behavior. The latter half of this chapter addresses these issues.

6.3.1 **Clinical uses of the term 'manipulative'**

Little research has been conducted on how the term 'manipulation' is used in a clinical setting, but what has been done suggests that people mean many things, all of which are negative.

- In one study, six different types of behaviors were labeled as manipulation by nurses, ranging from bullying, intimidation, and physical violence to building special relationships in order to secure clinician compliance to conning and lying. (Bowers 2002)

- In the Hare Psychopathy Checklist, lying and making false promises are distinguished from manipulativity, where manipulation is defined as deception used for personal gain, without concern for victims. (Hare 1991, cited in Bowers 2003)

- The Fallon Inquiry included, as manipulative behavior, patients who threatened to make official complaints if they were not treated the way they thought was right. (Fallon *et al.* 1999, cited in Bowers 2002)

Len Bowers offers a definition of manipulation that takes into account this broad array of behavior yet distills it so it has some clarity: manipulativity is activity that aims 'to achieve a desired goal (perverse or normal, symbolic or real) using deception, coercion and trickery, without regard for the interests or needs of those used in the process' (Bowers 2003, p. 325). John Gunderson defines manipulation as 'those efforts by which covert means are used to control or gain support from significant others. Typical ways include somatic complaints, provocative actions, or misleading messages, as well as self-destructive acts' (Gunderson 1984, p. 5).

Other researchers classify manipulation as a type of covert or indirect aggression, where the aggression is disguised (Kaukianinen *et al.* 2001, p. 361), and they define aggression as 'a response, the intent of which is to injure another person' (p. 363). Indirect aggression typically is circuitous, and the aggressor tries to 'hide his or her overt intentions to harm others by applying strategies, which disguise aggression in the form of discreet or malicious insinuations' (p. 363). Examples of covert insinuative aggression include the use of negative glances and gestures, do-not-speak-to-me behaviors, interrupting someone on purpose, imitating an employee's style of walk, expressions, or gestures in a derogative manner, refusing to listen to the other person, and hinting that the other person has mental problems (p. 364). One question, then, is whether manipulation is a type of aggression or other deliberately injurious behavior and, in particular, whether the behavior of patients diagnosed with BPD should rightly be conceptualized this way. But the more difficult problem is that the concept of manipulation has such broad meaning in the clinical lexicon and that it is not clear what behavior clinicians are objectively observing that should count as manipulative.

6.3.2 Uses of the term in the broader society

Here I want to pose examples drawn from non-clinical situations. Some of these examples are claimed, by the writer, to be forms of manipulation. Others may fit a definition of manipulation but are not called that. This section will illustrate differences in how the concept of manipulativity is employed in clinical settings from the broader society and present more puzzles about what sort of behavior should be called manipulative.

The first example involves the stripper and her customer, in which interaction 'is a complicated mixture of manipulation and control of emotions and communication' (Pasko 2002, p. 63). Lisa Pasko argues that strippers are experienced at managing the emotions of their customers in order to earn a monetary reward. They play two roles: sex object for their customers and impersonators of 'counterfeit intimacy' (p. 56). But how they play out those roles depends on the individual customer's needs, so skillful strippers are adept at 'reading' their customers. 'Knowing when to act seductive, when to remain still and simply be nude, when to shock a shy customer with a sudden revelation of nudity and when to be talkative, come from a dancer's ability to decode men's sexual wishes' (p. 58).

Prima facie, it may be right to characterize strippers as manipulating the emotions and desires of their customers. But this kind of interaction is importantly different from behaviors like lying and deceiving because the customer has come to the strip joint for the purpose of having his fantasies played out. The stripper and the customer are aware that the stripper is playing a role and that, to do so successfully, she must intuit his needs sufficiently to satisfy him. The customer knows that the stripper is working to earn a tip, although he brackets off that knowledge in order to participate in the game. So, this kind of interaction is more like socially agreed-upon moves people make in a given context. In other words, I am arguing that some forms of behavior that might appear to be manipulative involve complex negotiations of people in social roles or are entered into with an implicit understanding.

A similar case can be made for flight attendants. In a training program for airline stewardesses, the trainees were told:

> You think how the new person resembles someone you know. You see your sister's eyes in someone sitting at that seat. That makes you want to put out for them. I like to think of the [airplane] cabin as the living room of my own home. When someone drops in [at home], you may not know them, but you get something for them. You put that on a grand scale–thirty-six passengers per flight attendant–but it's the same feeling.

(Hochschild 1983, p. 105)

Hochschild does not identify this thinking as a precursor to manipulativity but does argue that stewardesses and other service workers are explicitly taught to manage the emotions of customers (and themselves). The flight attendant, for example, is expected to act pleased to serve the travelers and to experience pleasure from her or his job. But, as with the example of the stripper–customer interaction, I argue that managing others' emotions to gain an outcome one desires is not always manipulative. Travelers are not fooled by gracious and pleasant behavior into thinking that each of us is special and brings a warm glow to the flight attendant who serves us; this interaction, too, is based on social understandings of roles and norms for behavior in a particular context.

Neither in the case of the stripper nor the stewardess are the behaviors malicious or deliberately injurious. They are socially prescribed interactions that are entered into with tacit agreement of the norms of interaction in those exchanges.

Con artists are called manipulative, but their interactional relation is different again. What distinguishes this case from the examples of the stripper and the stewardess is that the con game can only work if the victim is ignorant of what is truly occurring. 'The confidence game is an act of trust development, fake pretenses and duplicity in order to acquire some kind of gain, usually monetary. The confidence game, like many acts of deception, is an assumption of power. ... The confidence person, or swindler, often enjoys the development and exercise of power over their victims, repetitively proving his or her cleverness and superiority' (Pasko 2002, p. 52). Con artists depend on deceit to fool their victims, and their explicit aim is to gain something from the victim that he or she would not otherwise have surrendered. This case does seem to fit the general idea of manipulation as bad means to achieve one's ends, but I will argue later that deception and manipulation are analytically separate concepts. For now, let me offer two more examples from the broader society that are a bit messier.

In a novel about a middle-aged woman having an affair with a young boy, the narrator says of the boy:

> It is pretty clear to me that there was a strong element of calculation in these little bursts of wistfulness and wonderment. By which I do not mean to imply that the boy was cynical exactly. Simply anxious to please. He had observed that Sheba liked him best when he was saying sensitive things about paintings and so on, and he was beefing up his moony ponderings accordingly. If this is cynical, then we must allow that all courtship is cynical. Connolly was doing as all people do in such situations–tricking out his stall with an eye to what would best please his customer.

> (Heller 2003, pp. 46–47)

Courtship rituals, although culturally varied, typically include the assumption that the other is showing himself at his best, downplaying or perhaps suppressing his bad tendencies, and attending to the beloved with an aim to please. Do people's interactions when entering into new potential intimacies involve a kind of manipulation? It depends. On the one hand, courtship is similar to the stripping and service industries in that it involves a tacit understanding of the rules of romance. It seems best viewed as a social negotiation that both parties know involves some exaggeration and some disguise. If Sheba likes daffodils and Connolly brings her a bouquet, most people would not see that action as manipulative. On the other hand, deception can run deep. Connolly could be posing as a lover when he really wants access to her money, or her younger sister. But then why not just call it deception or exploitation? Courtship *per se* is not manipulative; the context of the situation will determine how to evaluate an interaction.

The last example also makes this point. Recall that, in the clinical literature, one type of behavior that counted as manipulative was patients threatening to make official complaints if they were not treated right. But consider this type of behavior in another context. The United States has had a long history of non-violent strikes and other forms of protest over unfair labor conditions. For example, 'In the women's garment industry, as far back as 1910, workers have ceased operations without leaving the shop. Partly this has been done when a contract forbade strikes, the workers arguing that a mere stoppage was not a violation' (Lynd S and Lynd A 1995, p. 142). Protests and strikes occur when people experience injustice or a violation of their rights and other forms of redress are unavailable. When power imbalances exist and the more powerful party refuses to negotiate in good faith, the less powerful may threaten other actions such as strikes or protests. Are threats always manipulative? A threat to strike may simply be the next move in a frustrating attempt to be taken seriously. In our society, we do not ordinarily talk about threats to strike as manipulative (although employers might frame it that way). Furthermore, it's not clear that attempts to claim a right to be treated fairly should fall into the category of 'intent to harm.'

This example raises the question of why BPD patients who are similarly less powerful and need pathways to ensure fair treatment are called manipulative when they threaten to take advantage of those securities. On the other hand, Bowers (2002) argues that, while some complaints are justifiable and for good cause, others seem to be done spitefully or over trivial matters. He says that 'the formal complaints procedure can be very destructive, can cause much worry even among those who have only witnessed what it has done to others, and is costly in terms of management time, suspensions, illness and resignations at a time when nursing staff are a scarce resource' (Bowers 2002, p. 62). Putting Bowers' ideas together with the above argument, I would say that manipulativity in patients who threaten to make official complaints would not consist in the activity *per se* but in a cluster of other issues that must be viewed in the context, such as what a particular patient's motives are, what events preceded the complaint, how dysfunctional the patient is, and so on. In other words, the act of threatening to make an official complaint does not *entail* manipulativity any more than the act of threatening to strike does.

6.4 Implication for clinicians and BPD patients when the concept of manipulativity is employed

Considering these examples, I note considerable messiness in the usage and meaning of manipulation in broader society as well as in clinical contexts. I identify two problems in the use of the term 'manipulation,' then. One problem is that, even in the restricted domain of clinical contexts, the class of behaviors is over-inclusive. Research suggests that clinicians include under the umbrella term of manipulativity everything from bullying, intimidation, physical violence, building special relationships, conning and lying, using deception for personal gain without concern for victims, and threatening to make official complaints if they did not get a request met (Bowers 2003). With such a range of behaviors, the primary message seems to be a negative judgment – vague in content but powerful in effect. Clinicians use the term as a superordinate category under which morally wrong ways of interacting are included. But lumping all these behaviors together is not therapeutically useful because it doesn't allow for differentiation between kinds of behavior that vary among BPD patients.

Furthermore, moral wrongdoings (such as lying) *are* distinguished from other kinds of wrongdoing (such as being divisive) both in moral theory and in ordinary language; the action, intention, and type of harm done are part of the evaluation of what makes each action wrong, and the identifying features of each of these moral wrongs are importantly different. So, it is a mistake for clinicians to group all these behaviors under a general heading of manipulativity.

The second problem is that a mismatch exists between the meaning of the term in everyday settings and in clinical settings. Clinically, the term refers to behaviors such as lying, bullying, intimidating, demanding fair treatment, creating divisions, and corrupting others. In ordinary life, many similar behaviors are not called manipulative. Is this mismatch warranted? Are all of us more manipulative than we think – and, if so, what would that finding indicate about the ordinary person's mental health? Or are BPD patients being held to a higher standard of behavior and interaction than are others?

Most people occasionally deceive, are indirect about what they want, disguise their true feelings, and intimidate others (Goffman 1952). But BPD patients are routinely characterized – pejoratively – as manipulative. Why are patients viewed through this lens rather than seen as participants in an acceptable social-role interaction in the context, or engaged in a type of persuasion, or as making a move in a negotiation? How can we distinguish 'normal' manipulative behavior from pathological, especially with the apparent variations between behavior and usage?

Let me take the latter question first.

6.5 Two initial difficulties in evaluating putative manipulation

We might conclude that manipulation is a matter of degree: a continuum from 'normal *quid pro quos* of everyday social life' (Bowers 2003, p. 326) to habitual, deeply ingrained patterns from which everything flows. This move would require us to distinguish manipulative *acts* from manipulative *character*. The borderline personality, then, would have a manipulative character.

This move is too quick, though, because we cannot rule out the possibility that patients perform complex negotiations in their relationships with clinicians and that those interactions are socially encoded in the patients' view. The patient role is a core function of health care and, although Internet access has empowered some patients to a degree, the social expectations for behavior of those in the patient role are still that of subordination to expertise and authority, compliance, and a bit of humility. Patients who challenge the traditional norms of the role are seen as non-compliant and, in the opening transcription between Lotta ('Ms. A') and the therapist, as indicators of the patient's disordered personality. An alternative would be to consider how the patient is attempting to navigate clearly delineated relations of power and to negotiate shifts in social roles so as not to feel powerless and beholden.

Another approach to distinguishing between everyday and pathological manipulativity is to identify what forms of manipulativity are dysfunctional or maladaptive. Numerous clinicians, in describing the BPD's non-compliant, self-injurious, and manipulative behaviors, refer to such behavior as maladaptive (cf. Harvey and Watters 1998). To call BPD manipulativity 'maladaptive,' though, merely pushes the question back: Why, and when, is manipulativity maladaptive? If I am right, the behavior that is called manipulative in clinical settings is condoned, expected, or not even noticed in non-clinical settings; we need to have a non-circular way of identifying pathological manipulation. I return to this point later.

For now, let me address the second question I raised: Why *are* patients viewed through a lens of dysfunctional 'manipulation' rather than seen as participants in tacitly understood social interactions, or engaged in a type of persuasion, or as making a move in a negotiation? The reason is that clinicians are as likely to perceive manipulative behavior based on preconceived notions of BPD patients as they are to base judgments on clear and objective perception. That is, their perceptions may be based on stereotypes of BPD patients. For example, researchers Gallop *et al.* (1989) asked: Do patients diagnosed with BPD receive qualitatively different care from patients diagnosed with other [non-personality disordered] diagnoses? Hypothetical vignettes in which the only variable was the presence or absence of a diagnosis of personality disorder suggested that stereotyped perceptions play a crucial role in how the behavior of BPD patients are interpreted and responded to. 'The difficult behavior of the patient with borderline personality disorder is often seen as "bad" and "deliberate" rather than as "sick"... The schizophrenic patient, on the other hand, is not perceived as having this control.' (Gallop *et al.* 1989, p. 815). Schizophrenic patients are perceived as ill, whereas 'borderline patients ... do not meet the criteria of "good and attractive" patients. They are not perceived as sick, compliant, cooperative, or grateful' (Gallop *et al.* 1989, p. 819). The researchers conclude that 'the label [BPD] is sufficient to diminish staff's expressed empathy ...' (Gallop *et al.* 1989, p. 815). Nurses were more likely to give responses that indicated affective involvement if the patient's diagnosis was schizophrenia and were more likely to give responses that were belittling or contradicting if the patient's diagnosis was BPD. The researchers suggest that clinicians and staff may believe that BPD patients 'deserve' less empathetic treatment and that their diagnosis is 'bad' or manipulative (Gallop *et al.* 1989, p. 818). Research by Bowers returned similar responses: nurses were virtually unanimous that these patients are to blame for their behavior (2002, p. 84). They reason that, unless a patient is deluded or hallucinating, or confused or muddled, she knows what she is doing and is therefore responsible for what she does (Bowers 2002, p. 85).

This discussion thus points to three questions: (1) Are clinicians seeing something objectively 'real' in BPD patients? (2) Is that behavior best described as 'manipulative?' Given the pejorative use of the term when referring to BPD patients, it is being used to convey strong disapproval. (3) What is *wrong* with patients manipulating their clinicians and staff ? The second half of this essay considers possible answers to this last question and shows how moral values and values of psychological well-being are intertwined.

6.5.1 What is wrong with being manipulative?

Response 1: It depends on what we include in the category.

If clinicians were to have a more precise and widely accepted definition, they would apply it less frequently and less sweepingly to BPD patients. Let me try to focus the term by distinguishing it from a cluster of related behaviors that include coercion, manipulation, and persuasion. (By doing so, I am disagreeing with the broad scope that Marcia Baron (2003) gives to manipulation). The connected thread of these concepts is that each is used to produce belief or action in another. In other words, the superordinate genus is 'behavior that is used to produce belief or action in another' and manipulation is one of the types. According to Claudia Mills (1995), manipulation has the aim of effecting change in another's internal states; it works on our beliefs and desires – and especially our emotions – in an indirect way. Manipulation results in a person holding desires and beliefs that (a) do not grow in any natural way out of her previous beliefs and desires and (b) 'are produced in a way that bypasses all of her ordinary cognitive and affective processes' (p. 100).

Mills' idea is useful. If clinicians were to follow this understanding of manipulativity, only those behaviors that work indirectly and on the level of the other's beliefs and desires would count as manipulative, and many behaviors now counted as manipulative would be reclassified. But her suggestion of what manipulation is doesn't help us understand why it is normatively less desirable than what she calls persuasion. What is wrong with being indirect? And when?

If being indirect is the marker for what is wrong with being manipulative, we need to turn to means-ends analyses. The idea seems to be that being direct with others when trying to produce beliefs and feelings is better than being indirect. The sense of 'better' or 'preferable' is both moral and epistemological because indirect behaviors such as lying about one's feelings are typically judged as morally wrong as well as epistemically irresponsible to the other. A negative judgment of manipulativity is based on the norm that the means to one's desired end should be achieved as directly as possible while allowing the other to participate in rational evaluation.

While this seems right, reliance on such a norm is fairly superficial. First, it ignores norms for interaction where complex negotiations of social roles may appropriately demand subtlety and finesse. Second, as Douglas Walton (1998) argues, different dialogical contexts call for different interactional styles. Third, what counts as indirect or covert is culture bound. What are the underlying values that lead us to object to indirect and covert means of interacting? Since we sometimes do not object (we prefer the flight attendant to pretend he loves his job of serving us), what is it about the clinical context that seems to demand directness?

This leads me to think that Mills' definition is still too broad. I offer a working definition of manipulativity as behavior that exaggerates or dramatizes an emotion or need that the manipulator is experiencing and that targets a perceived vulnerability in the other (cf. Baron 2003, p. 44). It is typically indirect in that it highlights emotions or needs in ways designed to effect desirable responses in the other rather than asking for what the speaker wants without dramatizing it. She is not deceiving the other, exactly, but instead is 'making the most' of her emotions and needs. The speaker *performs* her emotional state in a way that makes it difficult to get a foothold in a more reasonable dialogue. The listener feels trapped because he feels that he has to take the speaker seriously even though he thinks that the emotion or need is being overdone.

This definition may be narrower than previous ones, but it is still not very specific. And it does little to advance our understanding of why behavior called manipulative is objectionable. Is it wrong – or dysfunctional – to exaggerate one's needs and emotions?

6.5.1.1 Manipulativity and blame

The difficulty for clinicians who work with BPD patients is that 'the concept of manipulation itself can become a scheme of interpretation' (Bowers 2003, p. 327) such that clinicians 'habitually seek out and impute manipulative motives to others' (p. 327). Perceptions of manipulative behavior combined with the strong feelings it arouses leads clinicians and staff to be less empathetic toward BPD patients. It is crucial for those working with BPD patients, therefore, to interrupt global assessments of manipulativity and critically to evaluate assumptions about what constitutes manipulative behavior. Furthermore, it is important to remember that feeling manipulated is not evidence that one has been manipulated. Manipulation has an objective aspect, and judgments of manipulativity should not be made wholly on a subjective basis. Nevertheless, BPD patients do tend to push people's buttons, and I think sometimes clinicians see behavior that is indirect and covert in frustrating ways. Consider the following brief case study.

6.5.1.2 Vignette

Ms. B was a 35-year-old disheveled, agitated, overweight single woman who appeared for her first clinic appointment. She promptly stated that she was grateful to 'now have a therapist,' and that she had needed one for 3 years. Even as the evaluating clinician felt uneasy about the role assigned by the patient, she went on to say she felt very suicidal. In response to the clinician's inquiries, she reported that she had been suicidal 'off and on for many years' and already had 31 hospitalizations.

> Clinician: What has caused you to become suicidal now?
> Patient: I don't know; what difference does it make? (now becoming irritated and defensive)
> Clinician: Has anything happened in your life recently? (Clinician is skeptical about the patient's lethality and hoping to isolate specific events that can be addressed but already feeling highly anxious about the patient's volatility and potential flight.)
> Patient: All I know is that I visited my parents and became very upset and had to leave. No, I don't know why. No, they didn't say anything. Yes, it's happened before, and last time I nearly killed myself.
> Clinician: What happened?
> Patient: I drank a quart of vodka, and then took any fucking pills I could find ... I would have been dead if my landlord hadn't noticed that the TV was on all night.
> Clinician (not convinced that the patient is dangerous, but still feeling coerced into suggesting hospitalization): Are you feeling that way again?
> Patient: I just want to get control of myself. If I can't, I'm going to slash my neck. This time I don't want to fail.
> Clinician: Would you like to go into the hospital?
> Patient: Yes, I need to.

(Gunderson 2001, p. 97–98)

Gunderson comments that this situation is a typical one for clinicians treating BPD patients and that the clinician will usually feel coerced, manipulated, and helpless (p. 98). Regardless of whether or not that judgment is warranted, clinicians are wary and easily aroused by perceived manipulation. A central aspect of such feelings of anger and entrapment is the attribution of choice and responsibility to the patient.

In slowing down a knee-jerk response to a patient who seems manipulative, we need to question the assumption that her means of reaching her goals are *deliberately* manipulative. It's a fundamental principle of moral philosophy that we don't blame people for things that are beyond their control. And our primary defense mechanisms such as projection, denial, and dissociation are part of our unconscious, so not subject to our will. Furthermore, the notion of choice and control is notoriously complex when it comes to socialization processes and learned styles of communicating. On what basis might we objectively determine that someone has *chosen* a manipulative style of interaction?

It might seem that I am suggesting that BPD patients cannot help what they do and so should not be judged so harshly. Then, the following would be the response.

Response 2: Manipulativity is not blameworthy when BPD patients do it.

The warrant for this view would be that this behavior is part of the dysfunctionality of borderline personality disorder.

But that's too simple. Responsibility for our actions is a moral attribute that we grow into as we gain insight into behaviors previously done unthinkingly or unconsciously. When we understand that we are behaving in hurtful or difficult ways and begin to see how we can change undesirable patterns of interaction, then we are blameworthy if we do not try to make those changes. In the therapeutic context, patients learn over time to evaluate behaviors as undesirable and acquire skills to intervene in learned maladaptive behaviors. We might modify the response to address that point, hence:

Response 3: Manipulation is not blameworthy when BPD patients do it, until their therapeutic development is such that they have within their power a foundation for self-intervention in undesirable manipulative behavior.

This sounds right. Such a view would at least require that clinicians not be judgmental and rejecting about perceived manipulation until they have adequately assessed the level of treatment and its success for an individual patient. But this response doesn't so much tell us why manipulation is objectionable behavior for patients to engage in, but at what point in treatment it can become a matter of blame rather than excuse. So, let me suggest other reasons why BPD manipulativity might be wrong.

Response 4: Manipulating others is wrong because it can lead to bad character traits (virtue ethics argument).

Our actions, over time, create the sorts of persons we become, and the character we have then directs our aims and goals such that our actions become informed by our character. If a person regularly uses manipulation as a method by which she achieves her ends, the long-term result is that it entrenches the disposition to manipulate others in order to get one's way. As a character trait, manipulativity is undesirable because it constrains and frustrates interactions with others and undermines trust. We might say, then, that the BPD patient has a manipulative character. This response classifies dispositional manipulativity as a vice.

But this move is too quick. As I indicated earlier, we cannot rule out the possibility that patients perform complex negotiations in their relationships with clinicians and that those interactions are socially encoded in the patients' view. Are patients manipulative in all contexts? Or is manipulation a sociological phenomenon that occurs particularly in response to clinicians? Are patients enacting a social role that is common among people who experience themselves as relatively powerless? Answers to these questions would be fruitful in evaluating manipulative behavior.

Response 5: Manipulating others is wrong because it is a wrong means to an end (means/ends argument).

It is a truism that, even when the ends are good, not all ways of achieving those ends are equal. To take one criterion of BPD – self-injurious behavior – even if the end of relieving stress, or feeling pain, or getting attention, is a good aim, concerned others typically do not want the patient to relieve stress or get attention *in those ways*. But what counts as acceptable means to various ends is normative, and I am reluctant to endorse 'indirectness' or 'performative exaggerated emotions' as wrong means without sociopolitical analysis of norms. And those norms will be relative to contexts, not universal norms. As I argued earlier, the context in which behavior occurs is crucial to the evaluation of that behavior.

Response 6: Manipulating others is wrong because it treats others as simply as means (Kantian argument).

The manipulative behaviors that we should judge most harshly are the ones where not only the means are wrong but also the ends are objectionable. For example, if the goal is to extract money with glee, as con artists do, then the means of deception is wrong and the goal of pleasurable exploitation is wrong too. Such behavior is wrong both on utilitarian and Kantian grounds, but here I highlight the Kantian view. Treating others simply as means to one's own ends, according to Kant, violates the Third Formulation of the Categorical Imperative. To exploit others in order to achieve one's own ends is to treat them simply as a means to one's own goals or as a being-for-others. It is morally wrong to get others to do things that they cannot rationally consent to or refuse because it violates our ability to be autonomous.

But it doesn't seem that BPD patients are treating clinicians simply as means. According to the more empathetic clinicians, when a patient is behaving 'manipulatively,' her *primary aim is to express her deep need for relationship* (Gilligan and Machioano 2002; emphasis added). Seeking relationship can, of course, fail – as when a man stalks a woman he desires. Stalking would, indeed, violate Kant's moral principles, as it imperils the victim's autonomy. But clinicians typically do not lose their autonomy in virtue of the behavior of BPD patients (unless the patient stalks her therapist, which then is 'stalking,' not 'manipulativity'). For BPD patients, efforts to seek relationship should be morally less troubling even if the way they go about it is less than optimal.

Response 7: Manipulating others is wrong because it violates norms of relationship (ethics of connectedness argument).

There may be another reason why there is so much blame going around when it comes to manipulative patients. BPD patients, when they do manipulate, are typically looking for relationship. In discussing a particular case, Gunderson notes that 'as usually the case, she as a borderline patient has trouble saying what is wanted. Unspoken is the fact that she wants concerned attention' (2001, p. 96). Gilligan and Machoian, too, suggest that what girls who are self-injurious or threaten suicide really want is 'the possibility of a confiding relationship' (2002, p. 323). It seems misguided to impute blame on someone for wanting attention and not feeling able to ask for it directly. And, as Marcia Linehan points out, some BPD patients are uncertain about what they feel and want (Linehan 1993, p. 230).

Norms of relationship, like other norms, are contextual. But at the core of relationship is the concept of connection, a quality that is both moral and psychological. I argued in Chapter 3 that flourishing is constituted in part by sustained connected relationship. Being in relationship 'is an ongoing process of making and recognizing reciprocal efforts to sustain connection and repair disconnections' (Potter 2002, p. 122). People are connected through the interplay of their feelings and their thoughts, thereby creating something new together that is built by both of them. This bridging experience is the 'connection between' (Miller 1986, p. 9). Manipulating another can disrupt the connection needed for a relationship to be sustained because when one person manipulates another, it is difficult for the other to trust either her own perception of the situation or the other's presentation of the self. Sustaining connection and repairing disconnections, then, is part of being in relationship in morally and psychologically healthy ways.

Many BPD patients experience great difficulty in maintaining relationships and, as a result, do not have the connectedness necessary to human flourishing. This loss, and the inability to know how to correct the problem, is one of the causes of these patients' great suffering (Zanarini *et al.* 1998). Manipulativity may be one way patients try to get these needs met; unfortunately, it is self-defeating.

The point that manipulation may be about relationship also might explain why clinicians react negatively when feeling manipulated. Extrapolating from a study done by Lawson (2000) on how it feels to be lied to, I hypothesize that being manipulated *calls into question the meaningfulness of the relationship.* Clinicians invest tremendous energy and time in working with their patients, including the development of a trusting and therapeutic relationship. When it looks like they value the patient/clinician relationship more highly than their patients do, it arouses resentment and anger.

I am partial to the last explanation because it captures the paradoxical quality of manipulative behavior while acknowledging clinicians' responses as some-times reasonable. The irony, for patients, is that the very thing they seek – relationship – is undermined by the means they employ to obtain it. Manipulating behavior estranges others over time: it suggests to the clinician that the relationship is not valuable enough to the patient for her to cease performing her pain, anger, and fear and to let it be experienced 'straight on.'

I am not arguing that the only reason BPD patients manipulate others – when they do – is that they are seeking relationship; people, including patients, manipulate for a variety of reasons. My aim has been to suggest what is objec-tionable about manipulative behavior, and I offered several arguments to that end. The point of the last response is to offer another explanation of why clini-cians would view manipulative behavior as wrong or bad.

Nevertheless, even this last response fails to address a crucial problem with judging manipulativity: the conflation of moral values with clinical values.

6.6 Morality and mental illness

As I have argued, meaningful relationships are central to living a flourishing life. It is hard to imagine a moral life without friendship, love, and companion-ship; personal attachments are part of morality as well as of well-being. And one indicator of mental illness is the relative absence of meaningful relation-ships, or difficulty in maintaining them. People diagnosed with borderline personality disorder often have unstable interpersonal relationships, and this difficulty is likely to cause the patient significant distress and suffering. This anguish is both psychological and moral because relationships are both psy-chological and moral. A link does exist between moral life and mental health.

For this reason, it is possible (easy, even) to let moral judgments about patients stand in for clinical judgments. If manipulating others is a dysfunc-tion, it must be shown to be one. I can imagine such an argument, for a dispo-sition to manipulate others can erode relationships and undermine trust, as I have argued above. When someone aches for relationship and connection but characteristically behaves in ways that prevent her from sustaining them, she is dysfunctional with respect to a vital human need. But I can also imagine a defense of behavior that is manipulative, for direct access to power and voice are not equally available to all of us, and manipulation may be a survival skill. If manipulating others cannot persuasively be viewed as a dysfunction, it should not occupy such a central place in the clinical literature on BPD. Three of the arguments against manipulativity that I examined – from virtue ethics, means-ends analyses, and Kant – are all moral arguments. For example, to call manipulativity a vice is to identify it as a moral failing, not a dysfunction. The last argument that manipulativity violates norms of relationship is both moral and psychological. But if manipulating others is a moral failing (and I think it can be), it should be viewed as just that: psychiatry should not be in the business of pronouncing moral judgments. Furthermore, I have argued that we cannot *a priori* determine whether behavior is manipulative or not, whether it is blameworthy or not, or whether it is dysfunctional or not and that these judgments require attention to the context, the persons involved, and their history.

Psychiatry is not free from values nor should it be. But the values that are endorsed must be carefully and reasonably chosen, not recycled from unexamined stereotypes or objectionable behavior.

6.7 Conclusion

Let's return to the opening exchange between Lotta (Ms. A) and the therapist. Does Lotta's behavior fit the working definition of manipulativity? To some extent, yes. She seems to have exaggerated her pain in order to get the therapist to pay her a visit. She wasn't particularly indirect, though. The discussion that the authors provide of the case raises the question whether the researchers are reading too much into the initial encounter. As I argued above, research suggests that BPD patients are perceived from the outset to be difficult and manipulative and that carers dislike such patients because they are not compliant and cooperative. The worry is that Lotta and the therapist are caught up in this dynamic. Another reading of the encounter is that Lotta is taking initiative to begin shaping the therapeutic relationship because she is anxious about it and does not want to feel that it is out of her control. In doing so, she draws upon not only dramatic ability ('You could be dying before you got any help around here!'), but also humor ('You must be either very good or very crazy to have taken me on') and directness ('By the way, I hate being called Ms. A.'). It does seem that Lotta is not following social norms for behavior in clinical encounters. Attempting to joke or asking to be called by her first name may be inappropriate in this setting, especially given the emergency call. But it is too quick to decide that '[a]lready in this initial interaction with Lotta's therapist-to-be, harbingers of the therapeutic challenges are evident' (Wheelis and Gunderson 1998). Inappropriateness in behavior suggests social ineptness, not necessarily dysfunction. And inappropriate behavior is sometimes the outcome when someone is challenging conventions and norms that are subjugating. Perhaps Lotta is actively resisting (in the political sense) the patient role as subservient, compliant, and subjugated. All this behavior could turn out to be dysfunctional for Lotta, but one encounter is insufficient to assess her. In order to know whether Lotta is dispositionally and pathologically manipulative, more time in interactions with her is needed, more context needs to be developed, and more attention to clinicians' perceptions and assumptions needs to be paid.

The question I have been addressing is whether clinicians are justified in taking a pejorative and judgmental stance toward BPD patients. While a violation of norms for relationship might provide an *explanation* of why clinicians react negatively to BPD patients, it doesn't provide *warrant* for sweeping labels of manipulativity or the negative attitudes that are entailed. Such attitudes do not satisfy therapeutic and moral norms that clinicians are expected to follow: namely, that clinicians need to develop empathy for their patients' suffering and distress. When clinicians view patients' primary character as morally objectionable, it's difficult for clinicians to feel empathy and for patients to either receive or elicit it.

Clarity and carefulness in applying the term 'manipulation' will aid clinicians in intercepting negative perceptions, a necessary correlate to being empathetic. BPD patients are suffering and need responses from clinicians that do not exacerbate their distress, and the pervasive attribution of pejorative and blaming manipulativity does not further their healing process.

Part II

Chapter 7

The trustworthy clinician

7.1 **Introduction**

This chapter begins an application of virtue theory to the therapeutic task of treating BPD patients. As I stated in the *Introduction*, I am not developing a treatment style; Marsha Linehan's dialectical behavioral therapy does a very fine job of that. Instead, I am pointing to some character traits that are important for clinicians to develop. This chapter focuses on one of the virtues and also serves as an introduction to Aristotelian virtue theory (in 7.3). There, I also take up meta-ethical issues that arise when discussing virtues. I argue that, according to Aristotelian virtue theory, virtues are both objective and contextual, a stance that I support. In each of the chapters in Part II, I suggest how to think of virtues as culturally embedded while still holding that there is such a thing as 'getting it wrong' about the expression of particular virtues within particular contexts. Chapter 8 discusses a virtue I call 'the virtue of giving uptake,' and in Chapter 9, I turn my attention to empathy as a virtue. Along the way, I relate the discussion to other moral and epistemological concepts such as 'world'-traveling, attentiveness, respect, and dignity. By discussing character traits, I emphasize moral aspects of therapeutic treatment that are under-discussed, to the detriment of BPD patient–clinician relations. Other virtues are undoubtedly important as well, but Part II provides a solid starting point in this important area.

The first virtue I discuss is that of trustworthiness. Trust plays an especially important role in clinical ethics; it's hard to imagine successful therapy if the patient doesn't trust her therapist. Yet most discussions about trust are sorely lacking in depth and clarity, and they typically focus on the wrong things. Analyses of trust, for instance, typically view trust as a kind of social contract or a kind of capital, and most discussions of trust that appear in the biomedical ethics literature focus on pragmatic issues rather than moral ones. Furthermore, most philosophical literature on trust approaches the topic from the angle of the potential truster who has to calculate costs and benefits. Such discussions provide inadequate grounds for clinicians to take seriously the corollary of trust: what it means to be trustworthy. My theory of trustworthiness, developed more fully in Potter (2002), addresses the shortcomings in the trust literature.

Starting from an analysis of what trust is, I show that being the person trusted entails certain moral responsibilities. Being trustworthy, I argue, is best understood as a virtue of character, where both feeling and action over time are constitutive of the sort of person one is. When we occupy an institutional role, such as clinician or professor, both general characteristics of trustworthiness and features specific to that role must be considered. After introducing features of trustworthiness, I indicate what trustworthiness would look like between a psychiatrist and a patient. Understanding the virtue of trustworthiness is particularly important in working with BPD patients, whose ability to trust others is damaged (Moskovitz 1996, p. 30; Meyer-Lindenberg 2008).[1]

Clinicians need to be critically self-reflective about the assumptions and ontologies to which they are committed. What clinicians bring to the therapeutic setting, for example in terms of theory, training, and status as a mental health expert, can impede the patient's therapeutic process. Again, I frame this problem as both an ethical and an epistemic one. Clinicians' moral responsibilities include the responsibility to be a certain kind of knower – one who engages the other – the patient – as a subject in his or her own right. And, clinicians' therapeutic responsibilities include the responsibility to help the patient become a reliable knower and to come to see herself as one (within a given patient's abilities).

7.2 **From trust to trustworthiness**

Trust, according to Annette Baier (1986), is a cooperative activity in which we engage so that we can assist one another in the care of goods. We trust others when we allow them the opportunity to take care of something we value. We all have to trust others, to some extent, because we cannot, by ourselves, take care of everything that is of value to us. Trust may be unconscious or unwanted; it may not be explicit, but it is possible (though not always easy) to say what, specifically, one is and is not entrusting another with. Most trust is specific to a person and a particular task or quality: I trust my research assistant Andrea to be timely in correcting my formatting mistakes; I trust my son Christian to take care of Grandma while I'm away – but I might not trust either of them to tend my flower garden. Rarely is trust in another global and total (though trust in a god might be complete and total).

----

[1] Meyer–Lindenberg draws upon game theory to compare levels of trust in BPD patients and controls and finds that the brain activity in BPD patients, specifically in the anterior insula, is abnormal. I have a number of reservations about this study but it is beyond the scope of this chapter to go into them.

Trusting another involves an expectation or belief that the trusted person has good intentions with regard to the care of something we value and the ability to carry through with what is expected of him or her. This definition of trust directs us toward an understanding of its relational nature: when we trust others, we stand in a particular relation to them with regard to some good which we are entrusting to their care.

Furthermore, this relation is one of vulnerability. Trust itself alters power positions (Baier 1986, p. 240): trusting others involves depending on them, being vulnerable to the possibility of disappointment or betrayal, and risking harm to self. This further feature of trust, in turn, indicates a moral require-ment of the one being trusted: being worthy of another's trust requires that one takes care to ensure that one does not exploit the potential power that one has to do harm to the trusting person. As we have seen with respect to BPD patients, the risk may be great that clinicians become inured to the vulnerability these patients feel: clinicians blame them, try to avoid them, view them as manipulative, and even may come to hate them. Even setting aside background conditions that make it difficult for some people to trust others, it is not hard to imagine that BPD patients, already wary and distrustful of others, may distrust clinicians.

In evaluating someone's trustworthiness, then, we need to know that she can be counted on, as a matter of the sort of person she is, to take care of those things with which we are considering entrusting her. When I trust someone because I believe her to have good will toward me, I have a belief about how I can expect to be treated by her that refers to *me* and that includes both her feelings and actions. When I trust my doctor to give me proper health care, and that trust is grounded in a belief of her good will toward me, I not only trust her to treat me well with regard to fair and ethical medical treatment, but I also trust her to be concerned for me as *this* patient that she is caring for and where her good will is personal and particular to me. We trust others more fully when we believe that they have positive feelings toward us not just as members of 'humankind' but in our particularity. This is because what we are considering entrusting to another's care matters to us – sometimes greatly – and when we believe that the other cares about us, we have more reason to believe that the taking-care-of will be done well. As Baier suggests, the best reason for believing that someone will care well for what we care about is that the person loves us (1986, p. 243). (If Baier is right about this, it is bad news for BPD patients, who are decidedly unloved).

I have taken as the starting point, then, that we trust others when we allow them the opportunity to take care of something we value and when we have favorable expectations that they will not disappoint our confidence in them;

the degree to which we trust will often depend on the extent to which we believe they have certain dispositions toward us and others, as well as the skills and knowledge specific to various caring activities. As readers know, trusting another may also be affected by a person's past experiences in trust and betrayal; children who feel betrayed by primary caregivers, in particular, often find it difficult to trust others even when others are, objectively, trustworthy. This last point is relevant to BPD patients, and I return to it in 7.5.1.

7.2.1 Limits on trust

Problems and possibilities of trusting relations aren't fully addressed by merely knowing what trust is. Trust can be cultivated, but it cannot be demanded of oneself or others (Baier 1986; cf. Reiland 2004). Secondly, sometimes it is clearly foolhardy to place our trust in someone. Given current societal conditions, where power, privilege, and oppression are realities of our political and social lives, trust is something few of us can afford to offer innocently and unreflectively. It is both morally and intellectually objectionable to trust in the face of strong reasons to suspect betrayal. So, it is not the case that morality demands that we trust one another, nor is it the case that trusting people are somehow more virtuous than distrusting people. Those views would certainly be incorrect; the reasonableness of trust depends upon particular contexts, so no such generalization can be drawn.

We are not required to accept the trust others place in us. At times it is appropriate to refuse trust – that is, to decline the invitation to be responsible for someone else's placing themselves or some good they care about in a vulnerable state. We might refuse to accept a confidence that a friend is wishing to divulge about her secret affair, for instance, because we wish to stay free of a net of deception and betrayal. Or we might refuse to accept the responsibility to be entrusted with the care of a friend's aging aunt because we already have many commitments and feel unable to take on another weighty responsibility. These refusals are not failures of trustworthiness, however; in fact, we may *exhibit* trustworthiness by clarifying what our limits are as well as by caring properly for those goods with which we are entrusted. For example, with respect to BPD patients, setting limits may seem like a betrayal to a patient even when those limits provide safety and security in the therapeutic context. Determining when the expression of trustworthiness should, in fact, be considered as such and when the expression of trustworthiness glosses over slights or betrayals is a delicate and difficult endeavor.

Still, living moral lives involves us doing our part to cultivate trust where appropriate. An ethics of responsibility and responsiveness to others requires that we do what we can to encourage the development of moral character both in ourselves and others, in our communities of participation, and in those with whom we come in contact (cf. Horsburgh 1960). Since trustworthiness is a morally praiseworthy quality, being considered trustworthy builds self-respect and encourages and sustains our trustworthiness (Horsburgh 1960).

7.3 **Crash course on virtue theory**

What is involved in being trustworthy and how can we determine who is and is not worthy of our trust? This question reflects a virtue theoretic conception of morality, which is distinct from either deontological or consequentialist moral theories. In virtue theory, the concept of character is central to morality (see Trianosky 1990; Watson 1990; Slote 2001). The question Aristotle is addressing in the *Nicomachean Ethics,* and the question he takes to be fundamentally important to *eudaimonia* (living well or flourishing; see my Introduction), is how we are to become morally good persons. Good persons are those who not only do the right things but also do them from an enduring disposition. These enduring dispositions or states of character he calls virtues.

Virtues are settled states of character that contribute to human flourishing. They are instrumentally good in that they are necessary for living a fully flourishing life, but they are intrinsically good as well (Aristotle 1985, 1097b). They consist in activities that express what is good and noble and that give the agent pleasure. Virtues must be exhibited, not merely possessed (Aristotle 1985, 1098b30–1099a6). To be virtuous, we have to have a tendency to express what is good and fine, using practical reason to decide what to do within a mean that is relative to us. Virtues are distinct from right actions because we can do the right thing accidentally or inconsistently, and we can do the right thing for the wrong reasons. Virtues, on the other hand, are dispositional; rather than getting it right in a haphazard manner, or only when we are in the mood, when we possess virtues we can be counted on to do the right thing for the reason that doing so will give us pleasure and because we love what is good and fine.

But virtue is not only a matter of being the sort of person who performs right actions but also of being the sort of person who has feelings appropriate to a given situation:

> [Virtue] pursues the mean because it is concerned with feelings and actions, and these admit of excess, deficiency and an intermediate condition. We can be afraid, e.g., or be confident, or have appetites, or get angry, or feel pity, in general have pleasure or pain, both too much and too little, and in both ways not well but [having these feelings] at the right times, about the right things, towards the right people, for the right end, and in the right way, is the intermediate and best condition, and this is proper to virtue. Similarly, actions also admit of excess, deficiency, and the intermediate condition.

(Aristotle 1985, 1106b15–1106b25)

As J.O. Urmson reminds us, Aristotle isn't meaning in this passage that virtue has two distinct fields – actions and feelings – but that whenever our actions are displaying our character, we will be manifesting one or more emotions as well. Actions embody emotions, Aristotle seems to be saying (Urmson 1980, p. 159). Or, as Nancy Sherman puts it, finding the mean requires that we act in a way that is appropriate to the situation, but it equally requires that we respond with the right sort of emotional sensitivity (Sherman 1989, p. 49). As with actions we perform, emotions are responses that affect both the agent and the observer, and the virtuous person cares about these responses; they matter in the way that virtue pursued for its own sake matters.

The virtuous person, then, exhibits actions and feelings within a mean. But the Doctrine of the Mean is neither a mathematical standard nor a mere call for moderation. Aristotle explicitly states that the mean is relative to us and, as W.F.R. Hardie puts it, the

> mean must be appropriate to circumstances including facts about the agent himself. The mean is not 'one and the same' for all (1106a32). The mathematical terms in which Aristotle chooses to express himself need not, and indeed cannot, be taken very seriously. It is a lecturer's patter. Do not imagine, he is saying, that finding the mean is a matter simply of 'splitting the difference' between opposing over- and under-estimates.
>
> (Hardie 1980, p. 135)

Because it is not a simple calculative standard, finding the mean requires that we exercise practical wisdom. As Richard Kraut says, we must consider the consequences that various alternatives would bring about for one's activity as an excellent practical reasoner (Kraut 1989, p. 332). But consequences are only one thing to be considered when aiming to reason well; I discussed the complexities of practical reasoning and deliberation in Chapter 4 and, especially, the messiness of figuring out when reasoning is done well. When I discuss the need to find the mean in given cases, I take it (the mean) to be a starting point for deliberation that motivates us to concentrate on contextual aspects of a situation while not allowing ourselves to slide into total relativism.

Philippa Foot explains that a person's virtue is assessed not only by his actions, and not only by his intentions, but also by his innermost desires as well. 'Small reactions of pleasure and displeasure [are] often the surest signs of a man's moral disposition' (Foot 1978, p. 5). This is why Foot argues that virtues are the expression of a *will* that is good, where 'will' is understood to include what is wished for as well as what is aimed at. Virtues engage the will, which is what distinguishes them from other things beneficial to our lives such as good health, and this also is what distinguishes virtues from skills and arts (which express a capacity but do not engage the will).

Another feature of virtues, according to Foot, is that they are corrective; they motivate us where we are deficient or bolster us where we are inclined to fall short of goodness. Aristotle recognizes that people have natural tendencies toward pleasure and cautions us to ward against it becoming too dominant in our lives. And Foot adds that 'there is, for instance, a virtue of industriousness only because idleness is a temptation; and of humility only because men tend to think too well of themselves. Hope is a virtue because despair too is a temptation; it might have been that no one cried that all was lost except where he could really see it to be so, and in this case there would have been no virtue of hope' (Foot 1978, p. 9). Virtues, then, help us overcome obstacles to living a consistently good life and guard against the tendency to get too caught up in a self-centered world-view with its attendant motives and inclinations. With respect to BPD patients, the corrective may serve to slow down clinicians' attitudes and reactions of blame and rejection and to develop empathy, a virtue I discuss in Chapter 9.

Virtues involve choice, (most) consist in a mean relative to us, and are concerned with both action and feeling. A virtuous person, then, is one who not only does virtuous things but also does them from an enduring state of character and in the way a virtuous person would do them (Aristotle 1985, Bk. 2). Linking character with the notion of an enduring disposition does not deny that we are situated selves. Aristotle acknowledged and attended to the situatedness of the members of the polis (but he interpreted differences [in equality, for instance] as detrimental to virtues [such as friendship]). Furthermore, the essentially social nature of character entails that, far from being static, it is in dynamic relation to self and other, both as a developing child and as a mature adult.

Our socially situated and shaped character is what makes us the sort of persons we are and gives us the projects and goals we aim at (Aristotle 1985, 1114b22–1114b2225). One of those ends is the care of those goods that we value; hence, issues of trust arise (especially if those goods are social in the first place as, for example, in the case of friendship). A trustworthy person is one who can be counted on, as a matter of the sort of person he or she is, to take care of those things that others entrust to one and (following the Doctrine of the Mean) whose ways of caring are neither excessive nor deficient.

What we have to go on, in this process of assessing the trustworthiness of others and becoming trustworthy moral agents ourselves, is our situated selves, our practices, our dispositions to be the sorts of persons we are and to do the sorts of things we do – our characters. But we are, in part, shaped by the social, political, and economic structures that underlie our particular relationships, and hence, questions about what it means to be trustworthy and how we can become trustworthy cannot be answered independent of how the state, institutions, and social relations are organized. Applied to the topic under examination in this book, trustworthiness and other virtues also need to be understood in the context of prevailing norms and expectations for normal and abnormal behavior. For example, as we saw in Chapter 3, womanly virtues include things that are detrimental to the flourishing of women, such as the reification of females' valuing attachment such that they fail to extricate themselves and their children from dangerous and damaging attachments. Virtue may be culturally situated but it is still possible to get virtue wrong.

The emphasis on character as the preferred moral theory is of value because it highlights particularity, context, relationship, and feeling – constructs that the prevailing moral theories of J.S. Mill and Emmanuel Kant eschew. Mill and Kant both envision the moral point of view as impartial, detached, and disinterested; this moral stance makes possible our ability to reason systematically and logically toward universal principles. But the impartial stance required by a principlist ethic discourages the task of revealing ourselves – our values, our beliefs, and our quirks – to potential trusting others, and so makes others' assessment of our character much more difficult. And it encourages us to think of others as generic human beings, an attitude that seems inimical to a therapeutic relationship. Impartiality, then, is morally, epistemologically, and pragmatically undesirable as a way to foster relations of trust between and clinician and patient.

Finally, I paraphrase Aristotle in stating that this project is but a beginning – for, presumably, the outline must come first, to be filled in later. If the sketch is good, then anyone, it seems, can advance and articulate it, and in such cases time is a good discoverer or (at least) a good co-worker. (Aristotle 1985, 1098a24). Because the mean is always relative to particulars, no theory will be able to cover every single case in advance. This is one reason why it is so important to develop intellectual virtue: so we can acquire the skills of good perception and practical reasoning needed to find the mean in a given case. Aristotle warns that we cannot expect precise rules to be discovered:

> But let us take it as agreed in advance that every account of the actions we must do has to be stated in outline, not exactly. As we also said at the start, the type of accounts we demand should reflect the subject-matter; and questions about actions and expediency, like questions about health, have no fixed [and invariable answers].
>
> (Aristotle 1985, 1104a)

Virtue theory will not – indeed, cannot – give us precise rules by which to live. What it does provide, though, is a vision of where we need to direct our attention and energy in order to become ethical clinicians.

Even though 'the mean is relative to us,' Aristotle does not think that morality is purely subjective. He argues that there is a natural world – that is, a world independent of our beliefs and desires – and morality consists in living in conformity with that world. For example, greed undermines the political community. Greed, as a deficiency in the domain of giving to others what is beyond our own needs, has a clear domain and a universality to it (cf. Nussbaum (1992) on the position that virtues are universals at a broad level). From these observations about the natural world, we can reason about the features of the good life, and these features are not subjective but are essential to all human beings. Aristotle argues that identifiable dispositional traits exist that a virtuous person would have and that provide a thread that runs through various situations and across diverse social groups. 'The virtuous person,' then, provides a moral point of view: when making moral decisions, we should make them from the perspective that a person of virtue would make them.

7.4 Some dispositional features of trustworthiness

In this section, I set out some of the dispositional features that a trustworthy person has and indicate their potential application to working with BPD patients. In 7.5, I work through two examples, one that is meant to illustrate pitfalls that coincide with many of the problems discussed in Part I such as assumptions and attitudes, and another that is meant to illustrate how an objectively trustworthy clinician deals with a deeply distrustful patient.

7.4.1 Features of trustworthiness:

(a) *That we give signs and assurances of our trustworthiness.*Trusting certainly seems risky in the face of doubts as to another's trustworthiness. As Baier states, reasonable trust requires that we have good grounds for believing another to be trustworthy and that we don't have reasons to suspect that another has strong operative motives, interests, affiliations, and loyalties which conflict with ours; distrust is reasonable when those conditions are absent (Baier 1986, p. 235). But these suggestions should not be taken as a gesture toward necessary and sufficient conditions for proper trust: the most that can be provided are heuristics. Trust is a practice that resembles induction: in trusting others, we always extrapolate from available evidence. In the final analysis, no decisive grounds for reasonable trust can be offered.

This point highlights the vulnerability of uncertainty involved in trusting others. How can clinicians cultivate trustworthiness in a way that attends to the power difference in the therapeutic relation and the sometimes strong distrust of the BPD patient, as well as to the inherent vulnerabilities that arise from the practice of trusting relations?

I draw on a passage from Rachel Reiland's book *Get Me out of Here*, a patient's memoir of her recovery from BPD, to give an example of how her clinician,

Dr. Padgett, gave her signs and assurances of his trustworthiness. Rachel had met Dr. Padgett while she was hospitalized. He decided to take her as a patient when she was released, and she had had one official full-length session with him. At the end of the session, he handed her a report from a personality test that was conducted while she had been in hospital. When she discovered that her diagnosis was BPD, she was furious with him: she felt betrayed, terrified, and enraged at what she saw as moral judgments about her. She accused him, swore at him, and railed against him hysterically [her word]. Two days later, she apologized profusely, expressing self-hate and pitiful remorse (a cycle that continued many times over). Here is Dr. Padgett's response, as told by Rachel:

> I'm not here to judge your behavior, he said gently, as my eyes remained fixed on the floor. I've committed to therapy with you, I want to help you, and I will honor that commitment. Maybe people have left you before or turned their backs when things got too rough. I won't do that. So long as you keep coming here, no matter what might happen, what you might say or do, it isn't going to drive me away. I'll be here. You can count on that. The only person that will leave this therapy is you: you will make that decision, not me. I'll be here for as long as it takes.
>
> (Reiland 2004, p. 60)

Now, Dr. Padgett is telling her that she can count on him, but his words and tone alone don't indicate that he will follow through on his claims. So, Rachel doesn't have a reason to trust him yet. Dr. Padgett acknowledges this problem:

> Trust is very very hard for you. I know that. I don't expect you to believe me or trust me right now. And I don't expect you to take me on my word. Talk is cheap. I'm sure you've heard plenty of talk. No, trust can't be proven by anything I say, but by what I do. You should be skeptical—questioning me at every turn. That's part of the process [of healing through therapy, I take it].
>
> (Reiland 2004, p. 61)

A patient who has a history of entrenched distrust, combined with being vulnerable with respect to the professionalism required in clinical settings, makes it more difficult for patients to assess the trustworthiness of clinicians (and others). As Dr. Padgett knows, it is not enough merely to *be* trustworthy; in order for therapy to be successful, the clinician must indicate to potential trusting others that the clinician is worthy of the patient's trust. Giving signs of trustworthiness is difficult when one is a clinician because maintaining appropriate boundaries is so important in therapeutic relationships. Thus, any discussion of trustworthiness in the therapeutic context must take into account the particular difficulties that arise for clinicians. As I stated earlier, holding and maintaining boundaries is a way to show that one is trustworthy because it tells the patient that she is safe, self-respecting, and capable of respecting another as well. For example, in a session where Rachel slaps herself repeatedly and does other self-injurious things, Dr. Padgett commands her to stop: 'This isn't therapy,' he says. 'This is acting out.' (Reiland 2004, p. 186). When he demanded that Rachel stop acting like a child, she did. In my view, this is an example of boundary setting that illustrates the clinician's trustworthiness in that he is taking care of the potentially adult and responsible Rachel by not allowing her to hurt and humiliate herself.

On the other hand, virtue theory doesn't deal with abstract generic beings; it requires that we engage with others in their particularity. The virtue of trustworthiness requires us to be willing to reveal enough of ourselves so that others can determine whether or not we are trustworthy with respect to something. Therefore, clinicians must find a delicate balance between maintaining appropriate boundaries and being open enough with patients so patients can begin to learn what they can entrust to their clinicians. But what counts as appropriate disclosure will depend not on an abstract code of ethics but on the persons involved, the length of time of the therapeutic relationship, the quality of relationship thus far, and so on. In other words, issues such as clinician disclosure of personal character traits that would illustrate trustworthiness must be particularized. Relations of trust are always inflected by the particularities of the parties involved, including cultural differences. This last point suggests that, in order to be trustworthy with respect to a particular patient, one must learn what sorts of signs and assurances would count as indications of trustworthiness in various cultural contexts. The disastrous cultural clash related in *The Spirit Catches You and You Fall Down* (Fadiman 1997) illustrates the failure of western medical practitioners to learn how to become trustworthy to the Hmong family, the Lees, with their very ill child Lia. Of course, many institutional, educational, and medical structures combined to give rise to the devastating effect of cultural divides – it can't all be chalked up to different ideals about trust and trustworthiness – but issues of trust were certainly a factor, one that it pays to keep in mind in discussions of the cultivation of virtue in psychiatry.

(b) *That we take epistemic responsibility seriously.* That properly trusting others requires an epistemic effort might be obvious; we have at least to know enough about a person to make warranted inferences about their good will and their various abilities as we entrust something we value to another's care. But it may be less obvious that *being trustworthy* also requires an epistemic effort. Being trustworthy requires not merely a passive dependability but an active engagement with self and others in knowing and making known one's own interests, values, moral beliefs, and positionality. This second requirement makes the Aristotelian point that we need to develop both intellectual and moral character in order to be fully virtuous: knowing well and being good are inextricably bound up with practical reason (Aristotle 1985, 1141b9–1142a10, 1144b14–1144b31).

To do so may involve engaging in critical self-reflection: How do our particular race and gender, for example, affect relations of trust with patients? In what ways do our values and assumptions impede being trustworthy to patients with some diagnoses and foster it with others? What are your attitudes toward BPD patients? Should those attitudes be challenged?

It will be a sign that we have taken seriously the moral demand of developing trustworthy characters if we actively engage in further reflection and dialogue about our assumptions of ourselves and others, the ways those assumptions underlie trust and distrust, and what we want and can expect from one another. A clinician can show her trustworthiness by engaging in critical self-reflection about the rejecting attitudes, assumptions, norms, and expectations that she may be bringing to the therapeutic encounter, as well as institutional (psychiatric) biases. Many of the problematic attitudes and assumptions that clinicians hold have been discussed in Part I of this book. Part of being epistemically responsible involves the next feature, described below.

(c) *That we develop sensitivity to the particularities of others.* To become trustworthy, one must attend to trust and distrust with respect to the various issues that different diagnoses raise. But this is not to suggest that a trustworthy clinician sees others only as members of various diagnoses. Being trustworthy also involves seeing others in their particularity. Sensing what others are counting on when they place their trust in us, and having a fairly good idea of who they are independent of our needs, projections, stereotypes, and fantasies, calls for moral struggle: clear vision is a result of moral imagination and moral effort (Murdoch 1970, p. 37). Trustworthiness cannot be found without grasping what it is, on the trusting person's view, one is caring for, and this involves an interactive and imaginative process of gaining some understanding of what the world is like from the perspective of that particular person. To do this may involve 'world'-traveling, a skill that draws upon epistemic responsibilities (the feature I outlined above). I discuss world-traveling as it applies to the mentally ill at length in another article (cf. Potter 2003), so here I just provide a sketch.

Marìa Lugones advocates the willful exercise of flexibility in shifting back and forth from one construction of life where a person is more or less 'at home' to other constructions of life. This willful exercise she calls *world-traveling.* To understand this concept, we first have to understand what Lugones means by a 'world.' A world is a kind of *experience* – where who we take ourselves to be is constructed through the concepts and norms, the language, history, and interpersonal relations of the inhabitants of that world (present living ones, ancestral ones, and even imaginary ones). For example, I may be constructed among African American activists as a fairly conventional white middle-class mother with a career, even though I may not understand or accept myself that way. 'I may be animating such a construction,' Lugones writes, 'even though I may not intend my moves, gestures, acts in that way' (Lugones 1997, p. 395). To world-travel, then, is to shift from one world to another, or to live in more than one world at the same time. Traveling involves a kind of shift in constructions of the self.

Lugones points out, however, that some people – for example, women of color – necessarily, as a matter of survival, become adept at world-traveling, whereas others – for example, white western philosophers – have less experience, less facility, less need, and less interest in traveling to the worlds of others whose constructions of us might be ones we don't recognize (or don't want to recognize). Genuine world-traveling is not a matter of merely acknowledging differences and honoring an abstract idea of plurality while implementing plans designed to improve others' lives as *I* understand them. To world-travel is to leave the familiarity of home. Being at ease involves being a fluent speaker in that world (in Wittgensteinian terms, knowing the language games); agreeing and being content with all the norms; being bonded to others through our loving one another; and having a shared history. World-traveling involves seeing both myself and another as I am constructed in the world of that person, that I witness her own sense of herself in her world. To do this requires that I learn to perceive differently. And this, in turn, requires that I abandon the comfort of the worlds in which I am most at home. (Readers will recall that I discussed the concept of home as it applies to the quest for safe relationships in Chapter 3).

World-traveling is distinct from empathy, although these two ways of responding to another's suffering are related. World-traveling is a methodology, whereas empathy is a moral and epistemological response. World-traveling answers the question of how I can *have* an empathetic response.

Empathy is a kind of perception that is cognitive as well as emotional and physiological. It involves the skill of place-taking combined with care and concern for the welfare of another. People often think of empathy primarily as a kind of emotional engagement, and it is that: to be empathetic, we need to be susceptible to others' emotions (what is called 'emotional contagion'). But the place-taking in empathy is also an epistemic venture in that it requires us to imagine and fantasize unconstrainedly, transposing ourselves into feelings, actions, and situations of others without identifying with them (Tamborini *et al.* 1990).

Much weight is given to the role of emotional contagion and imagination in learning how to empathize accurately. Yet even those considerations presuppose background conditions that may not exist: namely, the de-centering of the ego along with the norms, historicity, and linguistic practices that animate the center of that ego. Empathy, then, is an important moral response to suffering, but it is apolitical in a way that world-traveling is not. A richly sensitive understanding of another cannot be separated from the politics of difference. World-traveling may not give rise to empathy because, for example, one may never become enough at ease in that other 'world' to be anything other than displaced and frightened. But world-traveling, because it is a methodology and not only an experience or moral response, deepens and enriches the level of empathetic understanding of the other. Empathy is accurate to the extent that the empathetic person has engaged in genuine world-travel. 'Only when we have traveled to each others' "worlds" are we fully subjects to each other' (Lugones 1997, p. 401). The failure of love that can come from moral tourism is partly because we fail to see ourselves in others who are quite different from us (p. 393). By traveling to each others' 'worlds', we can learn to love each other (p. 390). This possibility can be the source of much hope for clinicians who have learned that BPD patients are sometimes hated.

The task for clinicians, then, is to learn to do this sort of traveling to BPD patients' worlds in order to understand how the world looks from the patient's point of view. As dispositional feature (c) indicates, when doing therapy with a patient, it is important to attend to this particular patient, not the abstract construct of 'the BPD patient.' It may be that most BPD patients are trusting their clinicians to help keep them safe, not to abandon them, not to mirror their self-loathing, not to automatically pathologize their anger, and so on. But clinicians should be wary of such generalizations, because they may miss important differences. For example, Marilee Strong (1998) cites patients' reports as to why they cut or otherwise injure themselves, and the answers vary widely: to experience control, to feel alive, to break through dissociative states, to communicate when words fail, to redefine the skin's boundaries, and so on. No one overarching reason explains all self-injurious behavior.

(d) *That we respond properly to broken trust.* How we respond, when we are (intentionally or not) complicit in the harms done to others, reflects and shapes our moral character. One expects a trustworthy person to care about having broken or disappointed his or her trust, and when the trusted person seems indifferent or callous to harm done to the trusting relation, it speaks ill of his or her character. Being accountable to others involves, in part, making efforts to bridge distrust and heal wounds when relations of trust are broken. When we have disrupted relations of trust, we ought to do what we can to restore that trust. Part of being trustworthy, then, involves trying to make reparations when we have harmed another. This restorative process, in the form of explanation, apology and, often, critical self-reflection and transformation, allows each person to address the harm and heal the damage. In working with BPD patients, clinicians are likely to be accused of betrayals when, in fact, they have acted in a trustworthy manner. For example, a clinician may hospitalize a patient against her will because the clinician believes the patient to be a danger to herself and the patient denies this. Even when the clinician believes her violation of her patient's trust to be a justified act that expresses her ultimate trustworthiness, she may need to do repair work with the patient so that the relationship can begin to heal.

(e) *That we need also to have other virtues.* I take the Aristotelian line that trustworthiness is part of a family of virtues that require the development of other-regarding or altruistic dispositions and that each of the virtues is necessary for the full expression of the rest. One such requirement, then, that is complementary to trustworthiness is that we have a genuine regard for the good of others.

Being trustworthy involves exhibiting the appropriate responses to others' pleasures and pains, suffering and joy. One cannot be fully trustworthy if one takes no pleasure in others' successes or if one is not disposed to share in the happiness of one's friend or fellow citizen. Likewise, one cannot be fully trustworthy if one has a disposition to ignore or overlook the harm and suffering of others. As Lawrence Blum argues concerning the virtue of compassion, when it is possible for one to relieve another person's suffering without undue demands on her time, energy, and priorities, the compassionate person is disposed to attempt to help. Blum notes that we wouldn't attribute compassion to someone if she sauntered by a fallen elderly man and left him on the sidewalk. (Blum 1987, p. 233–234).

Callousness toward others indicates that one hasn't developed the proper feelings toward pain and pleasure, the development of which is vital to moral education. Being virtuous, on an Aristotelian account, requires an intermediate condition of both feeling and action, and a person who generally feels little concern for the suffering of others or who is not moved to act to prevent harm and alleviate suffering seems to lack a quality that is vital to virtue (Aristotle 1985, Bk. 2). The requirement that we have a genuine regard for the good of others, then, asks of those who desire to become trustworthy that they cultivate feelings and actions that are properly responsive to harms done to others and suffering endured by others, relative to the mean. It requires of the trustworthy person not only that she be concerned about the possibility that she could exploit or harm others through excessive or deficient taking-care in trust and be disposed to non-exploitative caring, but also that she be concerned about the ways in which others are exploited or are suffering and that, even when she isn't the cause of the exploitation or suffering, she be disposed to do what she can to improve others' conditions of living. Thus, being trustworthy is integrally bound up with other virtues such as thoughtfulness, beneficence, justice, and compassion. The other virtues I identify as particularly important to being a good clinician with respect to BPD patients are the virtue of giving uptake and empathy, discussed in Chapters 8 and 9.

7.5 **An example to work with**

To fill out the theory of the trustworthy clinician, I discuss BPD in the context of a particular patient. (This example is also discussed in Chapter 6, but the focus is different; in that chapter, we examined the construct of manipulativity, and here, we apply the idea of clinician trustworthiness.)

A prevalent way for the past 20 years of characterizing the borderline patient is as a demanding, aggressive, and angry woman (Jiminez 1997). As we saw, Perry and Klerman pathologize patients' behavior for what seems clearly like a failure to comply with the social role assigned to women patients: Angry, assertive women, and women who resist expectations that they be especially attentive to social nuance, are defying social norms for femininity and are vulnerable to being considered mentally ill; such behavior, coupled with their own expressions of emptiness, aloneness, or identitylessness are taken as confirming evidence of BPD.

The intersection of gendered norms for behavior and norms for 'the good patient' can influence clinicians' interpretations of dialogical exchanges, to the detriment of BPD patients. This exchange takes place as a medical emergency the night before the first scheduled appointment between therapist and patient. I repeat the transcript in full so readers can re-familiarize themselves with this case:

> Ms. A: You could be dying before you got any help around here! My arm is killing me! This place is crazy!
> Therapist: Ms. A, I would like to introduce myself. I am Dr. Wheelis.
> Ms. A: Oh, no kidding! I didn't expect you. You're a resident? Interesting. You must be either very good or very crazy to have taken me on.
> Therapist: I can't tell if that's an invitation, a warning, or both [patient smiled at the comment], but we have an appointment tomorrow. Why don't we discuss it then. For now, perhaps I should take a look at your arm.
> Ms. A: No, it's okay, just a little bang.
> Therapist: Are you sure? You suggested that it was giving you considerable pain.
> Ms. A: No, it's fine, really. I'll see you tomorrow. By the way, I hate being called Ms. A.

Therapist: How would you like to be called?
Ms. A: Lotta. That's what everyone calls me.
Therapist: Very well, as you wish.

This exchange suggests that the therapist has taken steps to assure the patient that she is worthy of her patient's trust: she shows concern for Ms. A, willingly agrees to honor the patient's value of how to be addressed, yet sets clear boundaries (as BPD patients are said to need). On the face of it, it looks like the therapist hasn't given this new patient reasons not to trust her. But the therapist's own discussion of the case following this exchange suggests otherwise (cf. Chapter 6, pp. 98). As I indicated in the discussion of manipulativity, I worry that the therapist sees markers of BPD–manipulativity, efforts to control others, repudiation of socially accepted boundaries, resistance to socially approved conduct–that could be theory-driven rather than symptom-responsive. Here the focus of the worry is that, by seeing the patient's behavior as a diagnostic category, the clinician undermines the crucial bonds of trust that need to develop between Ms. A and the clinician. What she may not see, given the diagnostic lens through which she looks, is how the world appears – and how she, the therapist, appears – from the perspective of the patient. Quick to make evaluative judgments about Ms. A's style of interacting, the therapist neglects other epistemic and moral responsibilities.

Considering this exchange in light of the theory of trustworthiness, we can identify questions that probe deeper into clinician trustworthiness.

- Does the therapist have a background framework of critically examining the many negative attitudes and assumptions that clinicians carry about BPD patients?

- Is she careful not to bring negative attitudes into the encounter and is she prepared to challenge ones that creep in?

- To what degree is the therapist aware of her own position(s) of power in relation to the patient?

- Does the therapist give signs of understanding the vulnerability of the patient in the moment?

- Is the therapist concerned (both openly and reflectively) about what, specifically, the patient is preparing to entrust to her?

- Does the therapist provide a space for the patient to indicate what valued goods she is or may be entrusting to the therapist?

- Is the therapist seeking from this patient the sorts of knowledge she needs in order to take care of those goods well?

- To what extent is the therapist genuinely drawing upon other virtues such as empathy?

◆ Is the therapist treating the relationship as one of potential trust, or as a contractual or fiduciary relationship?

We don't know the answers to all these questions. But then, character isn't purely behavioral; it is a matter of feelings and intentions as well as actions. In thinking about what clinician trustworthiness would look like with regard to Ms. A, we have to know more about each of them and different ways the relationship might develop. Bonds of trust develop over time, of course, and it's not clear that Ms. A. was dissatisfied with this encounter. But trustworthiness isn't purely subjective: believing we are trustworthy — and even being trusted by some others — isn't evidence that we are, in fact, trustworthy in heart as well as hand. We are accountable not only to ourselves and to specific others, but to communities of others whose differing perspectives, burdens, and experiences sometimes elicit criticisms and concerns we ourselves miss.

7.5.1 **Another example**

The previous example points out some potential pitfalls in a therapeutic encounter. Here I offer a more positive one by returning to the relationship between Rachel Reiland and her psychiatrist, Dr. Padgett. This example is one where the patient's cognitive mistakes and dichotomous thinking lead to her distrust of even the trustworthy clinician.

Rachel is protesting a point Dr. Padgett made that she is still protecting herself by not allowing herself to be fully vulnerable to him. She asks, 'What in the hell makes you so worthy of trust anyway?' Dr Padgett replies,

> That's something you have to determine on your own: whether or not you are completely safe here. From our very first sessions, Rachel, I've never asked you to blindly trust me. I've encouraged you to be as skeptical as you need to be, to question me at every turn. Ultimately you have to be the one who determines if I'm safe to trust. When you are ready to do that, you will. But there's nothing I will say to try and convince you. Trust is given, not coerced.

> Great, I [Rachel] quipped sarcastically. 'Trust me.' Famous last words. Walk to the end of the plank with a blindfold on and just hope that somehow everything's going to work out. Hope that I won't be shark bait. No guarantees, mind you. Just 'trust me!'

> You're afraid.

> Of *course* I'm afraid, you fool! Who wouldn't be? Trusting completely is an invitation to be burned.

> In your past experiences, yes, he [Dr Padgett] said, ignoring my insult. Which is why you have to learn that trust doesn't universally lead to being burned. Sometimes it leads to feeling even more loved, safer, and more secure than before.

At this point, exasperated and afraid, Rachel exclaims, 'Do you have any idea what you're asking me to do?' And Dr. Padgett replies,

> Yes, I do know what I'm asking you to do. That's why I'm saying that you shouldn't trust me because I tell you that you need to, but because you've looked at the history of this relationship and drawn your own conclusions. It's painful and it's hard, but it's necessary. If it weren't in your best interest, I wouldn't even bring it up ... Take all the time you need. I'll be here for as long as it takes.

(Reiland 2004, p. 301–302)

By letting Rachel know that he is willing to be tested, that he invites skepticism, and that he is committed to working with her, Dr. Padgett sets the stage for trust to develop. He doesn't cajole her into making a leap of faith about him or about therapy. He is empathetic about her fears and distress. He is reassuring, reminding her that he has her best interests at heart. Perhaps most importantly, he says, 'I'll be here for as long as it takes,' addressing an underlining fear that Rachel has about being abandoned. In all these ways, he lets Rachel experience him as trustworthy, if she is ready and able to experience that.

7.6 Conclusion

This framework for trustworthiness started with an assumption that those who trust hold certain expectations and make inferences about whom to trust, and those assumptions are, roughly, right for many of us. But some people's mental distress is such that their cognitive capacities are greatly diminished. Although trust is a relation — and one where the act of trusting itself entails moral responsibilities of the trusted one — not all relations of trust take this form. That is, a patient may have no choice but to place into a clinician's hands something the patient greatly values. Clinicians still need to be trustworthy to those patients, because their cognitive impairment exacerbates their vulnerability. Trustworthiness, in these situations, is more like being the sort of person who would be worthy of a given patient's trust if that patient were able to make choices about whom to trust. Our feelings and actions need to be appropriate for that context even when the patient is incapable of forming expectations about future predictability or assessing others' good will. The relation of trust may look more like navigating upstream with no paddle partner. Yet one must travel responsibly, for both your sakes.

Chapter 8

Communicative ethics and the virtue of giving uptake

8.1 **An example**

Clinician (after greeting patient warmly): Let's start by looking at your diary card. [Therapist reviews the patient's daily diary reviewing suicidality, self-care, and periods of misery.]

Patient: It's been a good week—uh, two weeks actually.

Clinician: That's good. So tell me the reason you weren't here last week. [Inquiring about the second priority, therapy-interfering behavior.]

Patient: I overslept—had been unable to get to sleep, so finally I took a sleeping pill. I didn't want to, and I felt terrible when I woke up.

Clinician: That's a tough spot to be in. [Validates patient's dilemma.] Did you remember that you had an appointment?

Patient: Not until after I woke up. Then I knew I wouldn't be able to get here.

Clinician: How late did you sleep? [Assessing feasibility of her attending.]

Patient (irritated): I don't remember.

Therapist: You sound irritated.

Patient (calmer): Well, you make it seem as if I didn't want to come.

Therapist: Well, I'm sorry you missed. [Placating self-disclosure.] It's good that you got the sleep you needed. Now let's discuss ways to see what we can do to prevent this from happening again. [Invites collaboration on problem solving.]

(Gunderson 2001, p. 171; side comments in original)

John Gunderson uses this vignette to illustrate several ways in which dialectical behavioral therapy differs from other kinds of therapy. But it shows another important characteristic of good therapy as well – a moral and epistemic characteristic. In the last chapter, I said that, in order to be trustworthy, we also need to have other virtues. One of those virtues is what I call the virtue of giving uptake. In this chapter, I explain what this virtue is and why it is important for clinicians who work with BPD patients to cultivate. After setting out the virtue in 8.2, I point out where, in the above vignette, the clinician is giving uptake to the patient and how giving uptake benefits the therapeutic encounter. In 8.3, I set out five maxims that assist clinicians in giving uptake properly in response to self-injurious behavior, one issue that often arises in therapy that requires the appropriate giving of uptake. I then more briefly apply the virtue of giving uptake to patients' anger in 8.4. My expectation is that, by offering these applications to treatment, clinicians will be able to extend the virtue of giving uptake to other troublesome areas in therapy with BPD patients as well.

8.2 The concept of uptake

8.2.1 Communication and acknowledgment

J.L. Austin, in *How to Do Things with Words* (1975), argues that when we use words we are, in fact, performing actions. As Rae Langton puts it, 'Speech acts are a subset of actions in general, so there will always be some description under which a speech act is intentionally performed' (Langton 1993, p. 301). In Chapter 2, I explained that Austin introduced the concept of 'uptake' to characterize the role that the listener plays in affirming (or disconfirming) the meaning of a speech act. The idea is that some speech acts hold conventional meanings that require listener acknowledgment in order to count that communication *as* a speech act. For example (one of Austin's), we cannot be said to have warned an audience unless that audience hears what we say and takes what we say in a certain sense, say as an alarm, an alert, or a threat (Austin 1975, p. 571). Another example is that of promising: my promise to you can be said to be successful when you understand my speech act as one in which I place myself under obligation to you.

A proper response to another's communication is one that conveys an empathetic attitude toward the communicator or an earnest attempt to understand things from the communicator's point of view (I distinguish between uptake, empathy, and attentiveness below). But it's difficult for us to empathize with (or just take seriously) people who seem to be very different from us, and societal norms often discourage it, so reliance on patterns and conventions may impede, rather than facilitate, understanding. Many of the conventions of language are bound up with social conventions and power relations that can elide the voice of the disempowered, such as the mentally ill. So, giving uptake cannot simply be a matter of relying on norms and conventions of communication. In order to give uptake properly, the listener may need to do some world-traveling, a concept I discussed in the last chapter.

As we saw in Chapter 2, Marilyn Frye, expanding on Austin's idea, discusses uptake in terms of anger. 'Being angry at someone,' she writes, 'is somewhat like a speech act in that it has a certain conventional force whereby it sets people up in a certain sort of orientation to each other; and like a speech act, it cannot "come off" if it does not get uptake' (Frye 1983, p. 88). Uptake, then, occurs when the second party, listening to my speech act, reorients herself to me and the relation between us 'comes off' with an appropriate response. Women, Frye argues, typically do not get uptake on their anger because cultural norms allow men to ignore or trivialize it. While gender is not the only axis of power and so a straightforwardly binary account of language conventions in terms of gender would be oversimplified, Frye is right to identify patterns of relating that follow structural power relations. Relations between clinician and mentally ill patient – such as the BPD patient – are one such set.

In giving uptake, we still may not agree with the communicator; we can take others seriously and yet disagree. But when we take another seriously, we also take seriously the reasons that person gives for her actions and beliefs. To give uptake rightly, then, it is not enough simply to receive another's communication with the conventional understanding. We must try to understand what the world looks like *from the communicator's position*. This may require that we set aside preconceived ideas about value and meaning. For example, in Chapter 2, I discussed the importance of considering BPD anger as real-time anger and not just as primitive, defensive, childish anger; giving uptake to anger, in this case, means to take seriously the possibility that a patient's anger may be about current perceived insult or injury and may, in fact, be reasonable. But giving uptake to such anger is not necessarily to acquiesce to it. The first aspect of giving uptake, therefore, is to attempt genuinely to understand the communicant's point of view.

Of course, as deployers of signs, we don't always know what we're trying to communicate or our reasons for communicating something. Still, there is a danger in disregarding a communicator's explanations and drawing, instead, on cultural norms, or in assuming we know more about a communicator's meaning than she herself does. Listeners' responses to survivors of the Holocaust, for example, often clutch at a familiar lexicon that wards off the discomfort and fear that arises when hearing about an alien moral landscape (Langer 1991). When Hanna S. says that she survived through luck and stupidity, the listener protests 'No, you were plucky.' Langer argues that interviewers of Holocaust survivors override the speakers' interpretations of events out of a desire to preserve preconceived associations between victims of evil and heroic survival. In this context, though, familiar moral vocabulary and norms are irrelevant to a discourse that attempts to give voice to experiences of the Holocaust. The survivors are mining their common and deep memory about their experiences, thoughts, and feelings, but the interviewers have (or make) no cognitive or moral space to accept as real the things they are being told. The listener, then, fails to give uptake to the speaker by refusing to grant validity to the speaker's different system of signs. Instead, she explicitly discounts the interpretations given by the speaker telling the story.

We can extrapolate from Langer's analysis to a communicative ethic for clinicians who work with BPD patients. We have few, if any, language conventions to lead us through discourse about self-injury, for example, in a way that preserves the integrity of the communicator. And without conventions that are appropriate to the specific participants of a conversation to map our way, most hearers fall back on familiar conventions rather than chart new territory.

Another aspect of giving uptake, then, is that one doesn't impose interpretations and meanings that the (other) communicator is unwilling to receive except through coercion. People in positions of authority (parents, teachers, clinicians) can put pressure on others to acquiesce to their interpretations, and giving uptake rightly requires that we guard against such tendencies. Clinicians, among others, have the ability to silence the communications of the less powerful, and one effective way to do that is to stop a communication from counting as the action it was intended to be (Langton 1993). In other words, reliance on the conventions of one's own culture, place, and time may skew a listener's ability to give uptake to the communicator. It is true that, in trying to give uptake properly – and by holding meanings open rather than closing them off – a clinician may be left with little common ground by which she can receive and understand another's communications, and that experience can be quite disconcerting – frightening, even. But it is my belief that the communicative struggle, in this sort of situation, is integrally bound up with being an ethical clinician. Genuine understanding is not easy to come by, and we should expect it to call for moral, as well as epistemic, effort.

8.2.2 Giving uptake as a virtue

This broader way of framing uptake is situated in virtue theory. The virtue of giving uptake contributes to the flourishing of individuals and society and, as such, is important to understand more fully. The reasons for this will involve understanding how failure to give others uptake affects those others and thus can become a vice. I set out the deficiency in giving uptake shortly, but first let me situate uptake as a virtue more specifically. The issue here is whether or not the virtue of giving uptake really is a separate and distinct virtue.

As discussed in the previous chapter, most of the virtues have a scope by which they can be identified. The scope of courage is feelings of fear and confidence about frightening things; the scope of temperance is bodily pleasures and pains of touch and taste. The scope of the virtue I call 'the disposition to give uptake rightly' is dialogical responsiveness and openness in the context of plurality and power relations. Calling for us to be responsive and open to the differences and vulnerabilities of others may seem like I am merely invoking the longstanding moral concept of respect. But I am not. The scope of respectfulness might be something like attitudes about the worth of others. But giving uptake is not the same as being respectful. For one thing, I am not convinced that respectfulness is a virtue, if by 'respect' we mean granting others an intrinsic moral worth or value. Respect, then, would be something we should always grant others – in which case it wouldn't admit of an excess. Having a respectful attitude might still be necessary to the full expression of the virtue of being the sort of person who gives uptake rightly. But one may be respectful and, say, detached and disengaged in ways that leave the other feeling not quite heard or understood. So, however we classify respectfulness, a disposition to be respectful and a disposition to give uptake are distinct sorts of things.

Giving uptake involves a kind of respectfulness but is more than merely being respectful; it requires being attentive. Perhaps attentiveness could be a virtue, with its scope as perception of particulars and universals, or of details and unity. A deficiency of attentiveness would manifest itself in a tendency not to notice important details or to overlook the particulars of situations, whereas an excess of attentiveness would manifest itself in a tendency toward slavishness when it comes to details or an obsession with pinning down the particulars of a case at the expense of moving on to action – or something like that. I don't know whether or not attentiveness qualifies as a virtue. But if I am right about the scope of attentiveness, that scope is different from the scope of our virtue. And one can be attentive and yet miss the mark when it comes to giving uptake: people who tend to be good at one or the other are not necessarily concerned with the same things. For example, suppose a junior faculty in a psychiatry department asks for more patients and, hence, more responsibility, and her chair responds by assigning her 4 hours per day seeing patients and being the attending on rounds every morning (this in addition to department expectations that its faculty be actively involved in research and publishing). We might say that the chair of her department attended to her request – but responded with an exaggerated increase in responsibility, an increase that sets up the junior faculty for extreme stress or failure. The chair may have attended to her request, but did not give uptake to the spirit of it.

Empathy does seem like a likely candidate for being a virtue (although I will postpone an argue for it until the next chapter). Furthermore, it seems clear that, in order to cultivate a disposition to give uptake rightly, we must sometimes be empathetic in that we must try to understand how the other person sees things and experiences things from her point of view. But just because we must sometimes call upon one virtue in order to rightly exhibit another, it doesn't follow that those virtues ultimately collapse into one. The scope of empathy is distinctly different from that of the disposition to give uptake rightly: the virtue of empathy is concerned with cognitive and emotional perspective-taking of others as a response to another's distress, while the virtue of being the sort of person who gives uptake rightly is concerned with dialogic interactions in a pluralistic and unequal society. Clinicians and the rest of us need both virtues but they are distinct from one another.

8.2.3 Giving uptake as a dispositional feature of living a good life

All of us need to cultivate the virtue of giving uptake because the virtues in general are central to being a good person and to living a good life. Living a good life is not only an individual task; we need to help bring about the conditions for a good life for others as well. Virtue is social and communal, and living well is not just a goal for you or me, but for all of us together. Giving uptake is a crucial corrective to our tendency to be overly committed to prevailing norms and conceptual schemes. Being entrenched in a conceptual scheme or cultural milieu impedes our ability to communicate across differences, to expand our body of knowledge, and to foster democratic practices.

Clinicians, too, have an obligation to become the sorts of persons who will give uptake rightly. The primary obligation of clinicians, as for all medical practitioners, is to promote health and/or healing. To that end, professional codes of ethics charge clinicians with a duty to uphold values common to all medical practice, including values of respect, autonomy, dignity, benevolence, and non-exploitation. These values are important in that they set constraints on clinician/patient interactions so that relief from patient suffering and distress is facilitated as much as possible and not exacerbated or frustrated by a damaging therapeutic relation. These values and duties of medical practice are part of a larger moral landscape in which we recognize that all human beings have certain basic needs that must be met in order to live a life of minimum suffering and that some of those needs are in the moral domain. Most clinicians, I believe, are committed to professional standards of ethics. But, because we are culturally shaped, clinicians do not come to encounters unmediated. All of us perceive, reason, and evaluate through conceptual schemes that are embedded in socially situated norms. So, for clinicians to fully embody the values and commitments of medical practice, they will need to extend their ethical framework. Learning to give uptake is an instance of ways that clinicians need to stretch themselves morally and, because uptake is a virtue, it is part of what is involved in living well.

Clinicians need to give uptake to BPD patients, then, because it is part and parcel of treating others with respect and dignity (although, again, giving uptake does not reduce to treating others with respect and dignity). What clinicians need to give uptake about is the patient's perspective on her self-injurious acts, or her deliberative or impulsive decisional processes, or her anger, and so on. For example, as I discussed in Chapter 5, it is particularly difficult to understand self-injurious behavior and to know how to situate it in relation to other body modifications. When confronted with patients who self-injure, clinicians are in need of a corrective to the tendency to interpret *a priori* the meanings of such significations. Without the virtue of giving uptake, clinicians run the risk of silencing or distorting the communications of their patients (if they are, indeed, communications; I leave open the possibility that they sometimes are not). And silencing or distorting patient communications impedes treatment.

There is a second reason that clinicians are obligated to develop ethical responses to BPD patients by cultivating a virtue to give uptake, and that reason has to do with the relation of uptake to trust. Noting that a central component of any ethic is communicative, I point out that failure to give uptake can impede patient trust in the clinician. Good communication both requires and fosters trust, and trust is a crucial moral dimension of the therapeutic relationship. Patients are vulnerable to the power, knowledge, and expertise that come with being a clinician and may be concerned about being misunderstood or interpreted in ways they disagree with. Giving uptake is also morally important, then, because it fosters trust when patients experience their clinicians as sensitive to the vulnerability of their patients; being trustworthy, because it is nonexploitative and nondominating, facilitates therapy. But it would be a mistake to cast trust in purely instrumental terms. While it is true that proper trust may foster healing, being trustworthy is intrinsically good. Like friendship, trustworthiness needs no further justification, even though benefits may derive from it. It is also a mistake to construe therapeutic interests as separate from ethical ones. Both are concerned with helping others live as flourishing a life as possible. When aims conflict, therapeutic healing must build into the relationship a way to mend broken trust and restore moral equality (cf. Chapter 7 here; also Potter 2000).

The third reason for clinicians to take seriously the claim that a good clinician gives uptake to her patients is an epistemic one. Responsible knowers make efforts to perceive and to understand correctly. To the extent that our own conceptual schemas inhibit our ability to grasp meanings other than ones we are already prepared for, we may miss important truths. Clinicians, because they are trained to perceive pathologies and to interpret patients' behavior in ways that are consistent with prevailing norms for femininity, health, rationality, and propriety, may inadvertently impose interpretations on their clients. To do this, though, runs the risk of ending up with mistaken belief. In order to be a good healer, the clinician must have accurate knowledge. And to gather correct knowledge, the clinician will need to listen to the patient in ways that allow for new knowledge to emerge.

Cultivating the virtue of giving uptake, then, can facilitate clinician understanding of the difficult and complex behaviors engaged in by people diagnosed with BPD. This virtue is only one among many that clinicians need in order to treat patients in a therapeutically and ethically grounded manner. Compassion, integrity, justice, intellectual virtue, and others are also central to being a healer and therapist. Virtues are not the special provenance of clinicians, either: we all need the virtues. It is also true that being virtuous will not, in itself, heal the mentally ill. Patients diagnosed with BPD who self-injure, for example, may need to form contracts, be prescribed medications, and so on. But part of knowing how best to treat a particular BPD patient is coming to an understanding of what their behaviors mean to them, and to do that requires an ethics of communication, a central feature of which is the virtue of giving uptake.

As a virtue, giving uptake is a responsibility that is not equally and always binding upon us. Whether or not one is obligated to give uptake to another depends on each party's relation to power, to each other, to the content of speech, and so on. Being trustworthy often involves knowing how and when to give uptake, so we often find that these two virtues might be said to go together. Indeed, it is difficult to imagine a person who is fully trustworthy yet lacks the virtue of being able to give uptake rightly.

8.2.4 The extremes in giving uptake

8.2.4.a Theoretical underpinnings and the vice of deficiency: the relation of giving uptake to claim-making

To see why we should consider a deficiency in giving uptake as a potential vice, let's examine what happens when one is not given uptake (keeping in mind that one or two deficient actions do not a vice make, any more than repeated acts of appropriately giving uptake guarantee that a virtue is being expressed). The general idea I will argue for is that the failure to give uptake undermines trust and diminishes flourishing. The discussion here takes up the more general concept of vices in giving uptake; the relevance to BPD treatment is articulated later.

The first point is that a society in which individuals can flourish is one where the claiming of rights is possible, and receiving uptake is necessary to claiming. I am likening claiming to warning, promising, and marrying: claiming is an illocutionary act that doesn't come off unless there is uptake. Another way of putting the point is this: claiming cannot come off unless the audience is trustworthy with respect to the kind of listening and responsiveness that claiming requires. While the concept of making claims against others may only be one aspect of BPD behavior – especially found in anger as a response to perceived insult or injury – it is a way of understanding why a failure to give uptake is such a serious moral infraction. Readers should consider this section primarily to set up a theoretical framework for understanding the repercussions of having a dispositional deficiency in giving uptake.

One mark of powerlessness is an inability to perform speech acts that we might want to perform (Langton 1993, p. 314). One way this might happen is at the level of locution itself, where one is unable to make utterances. Another way is when one speaks but doesn't get the desired results; Langton calls this perlocutionary frustration. The third way is through 'illocutionary disablement,' where one utters words but doesn't get the desired result and it isn't recognized as the action one performed. This is a kind of silencing that occurs when an utterance is prevented from counting as the act it was intended to be.

A community or society that doesn't give uptake to claims thwarts the wellbeing of (at least some) members of that community and opens the door to other detrimental effects to the overall citizenry as well. Joel Feinberg shows, by asking readers to imagine a world called Nowheresville that does not have the concept of rights, that 'the activity of claiming, as much as any other thing, makes for self-respect and respect for others, gives sense to the notion of personal dignity, and distinguishes this otherwise morally flawed world from the even worse world of Nowheresville' (Feinberg 1970). And when a community or society fails to give sufficient weight to values of mutual respect and dignity, the social trust that holds groups together is undermined.

To fill out this idea, I return to Frye's argument that (most) men are socialized to respond to women's anger with dismissal. Refusing, on the basis of gender, to take seriously a woman's claims that an injustice has been done or a right violated is to reduce her status to membership in a class, and then to use that classification to justify ignoring those claims. But the act of claiming ought not be dealt with in this manner. To ignore someone's claims against someone on the basis of group membership is both morally and legally objectionable: it is the nature of claiming that each person is entitled to have her or his claims acknowledged at least to the degree that it is determined whether there is a legitimate claim to be investigated.

To affirm or deny that a right has been violated, it first must be acknowledged that a claim has been made. A claim may, in fact, turn out to rest on a mistake. But in some cases, the hearer refuses to acknowledge that an act of claiming has even occurred. The hearer fails to recognize the act, and the claiming is not given uptake. From the perspective of the hearer, nothing is claimed. And if nothing is acknowledged as having been claimed, then the question of whether or not a right has been violated simply doesn't get raised. The fact that claiming requires uptake in order for it to count as a speech act suggests that, in societies with systematic injustices encoded by linguistic conventions and discourses of power, many individuals' rights are likely to be threatened.

This is not to propound a simple equation of claims with rights. Feinberg notes that there is a *prima facie* sense of 'claim' which consists in acknowledging that one is entitled to a fair hearing and consideration – that the audience grants minimum plausibility that the speaker has a right to x without yet establishing that one has a right to x. But Feinberg also says that 'having a claim consists in being in a position to claim' – which position is not always recognized even when minimum plausibility ought, objectively speaking, to be granted (Feinberg 1970).

That is, structural injustices sometimes impede members of nondominant groups from being recognized as meeting *prima facie* conditions for claiming. Deciding whether or not to give uptake to a person's claims on the basis of membership of subjugated groups is both a symptom of oppression and an act of oppression.

> The ability to perform speech acts of certain kinds can be a mark of political power. To put the point crudely: powerful people can generally do more, say more, and have their speech count for more than can the powerless. If you are powerful, there are more things you can do with your words .... If you are powerful, you sometimes have the ability to silence the speech of the powerless ... But there is another, less dramatic but equally effective, way. Let them speak. Let them say whatever they like to whomever they like, but stop that speech from counting as an action. More precisely, stop it from counting as the action it was intended to be.
>
> (Langton 1993, pp. 298–299)

Consistently not giving uptake may be wrong because not to give at least *prima facie* credence to another's utterance is to treat that person as less than fully human: it is to say that, where that person is concerned, I don't have to consider his or her needs, views, claims, or emotions. Trust is diminished when an act of claiming is ignored as an action to be grappled with because a refusal to acknowledge the act as one of claiming calls into question the good will of the other to care for things the speaker values.

The link between this cluster of concepts – uptake, rights, and humanity – comes in with the concept of dignity. Dignity, as Bernard Boxill explains, is 'the sense that one's manifest humanity makes one manifestly worthy of one's human rights' (Boxill 1992, p. 197). Dignity functions here as a moral concept that is at once individual and communal. Robin Dillon states that 'as various declarations of human rights affirm, the equality of human dignity is taken to be the basis of the equal moral rights that all persons have as persons, independently of social law, custom, convention, and agreement' (Dillon 1995, p. 22). Failure to give uptake, then, (for example, when someone's speech act is that of claiming that a right has been violated) can be an assault on the speaker's dignity.

Presumably we can recover from the occasional assault on our dignity. But power relations render it more likely that the actual distribution of assaults on dignity falls regularly and consistently to the disempowered. A social climate where a group of people come to expect a lack of uptake on claims, coupled with assaults on one's dignity when one attempts to get uptake, eventually can undermine even the most resilient of folks. An environment like that is clearly not one for flourishing. Both the individuals themselves and society overall are diminished when dignity is threatened or lost. Furthermore, a society where claiming and giving uptake are activities that fall along power lines is less likely to progress toward the virtue of justice: to create and sustain a just society, claiming and giving uptake must be an ongoing practice in which a plurality of voices can and do participate. Finally, both localized and societal trust is impeded and distrust fueled when linguistic conventions lead to the lack of uptake.

Failure to give uptake can also be seen to be a potential vice if we consider not just an assault on one's dignity but on one's deepest psychological self. An example of this is found in Langer's *Holocaust Testimonies* (although his focus isn't on claiming). Langer, in his analysis of interviews with Holocaust survivors, argues that their selves and their memories are fragmented as a result of their wartime experiences (1991). Interviewers were ostensibly (and probably earnestly) seeking understanding of those experiences but, because they failed to give uptake, their good intentions turned out to be both self-and other-alienating.

The absence of uptake and experiences of others' untrustworthiness can give rise to rage in the speaker. It makes most people frustrated and angry to be ignored or misunderstood, or to have one's words trivialized or exaggerated. And rage can lead to violence: consider how the failure of the legal system to give uptake to Black males' reports of police brutality eventually led to collective outrage at injustice, voiced through rioting in cities across the United States after the Rodney King verdict. When individual speech acts are not given uptake (for example, when individual claims against the police force are ignored), collective activity is more likely to be emphatic, even violent, in increasing attempts to obtain that uptake. It seems clear that it would be better (in terms of constructive efforts toward a just society) for court systems and police departments to have given uptake earlier on. That is to say, one reason that not giving uptake should be a cause for concern is that it is one of the causes of the increase in violence in society which, in turn, diminishes the quality of life for citizens. Another reason to think that the failure to give uptake undermines trust and is detrimental to flourishing and, hence, is a potential vice is that it may silence the speaker. Uptake is not just a matter of receiving public recognition of various speech acts; part of the problem of institutionalized speech is that persons in nondominant groups don't have equal access to institutionalized speech.

Here we may find the relevance of the vice of deficiency to BPD patients. Many patients experience themselves as not being taken seriously, as not having a voice worth listening to, of being viewed as manipulative or of having an overdeveloped sense of entitlement. All of these self-perceptions fit neatly within an environment where others do not give them uptake. Anger, already suspect, may give rise to more anger; big anger combined with already-blaming and pejorative attitudes from clinicians diminishes clinician empathy and a healing climate.

8.2.4.b The extremes of giving uptake: giving uptake to excess

The responsibility to give uptake should not be understood as a requirement on demand: like trustworthiness, although I am morally bound to exhibit it, there is a right time, a right place, a right way, and so on. Since giving uptake is a move in a dialogue, and participants in dialogue have different social positions, histories, perspectives, and relationships of their own, no set rule can be established that can be applied across the board. And our responsibility to give uptake has to be balanced with other commitments, time constraints, and so on. For another thing, there may be encounters in our lives in which it would be downright dangerous to give uptake to an utterance (for instance, if I am walking home alone late at night and a stranger tries to make conversation with me).

But someone may, over time, develop a disposition to give uptake excessively. What would this look like? I can imagine two ways in which such a character trait would show up.

First let's return to the idea that the virtue we are considering – that of being the sort of person who gives uptake rightly – requires that one give uptake toward the right people, at the right time, in the right way, and so on. Now, one may, instead, develop a tendency always to give uptake to certain people such as authority figures or to an important person in one's life. When the excessive uptaker is faced with decisions or asked to voice opinions, she not only consults those others for advice but also takes their point of view to be the correct point of view without trying to differentiate her own beliefs from theirs or assessing ideas autonomously. As a disposition, this would be a deficiency because the person would not be in the habit of thinking for herself, and this habit would undermine her ability to be a good practical reasoner. Instead, she would listen so carefully to others and take seriously their views to the detriment of discerning for herself what is good and fine and pleasurable. Listening to others' advice and views to the exclusion of the development of one's own voice also calls one's trustworthiness in more general matters into question. How can others be confident that we can be counted on to take care of what is valuable to them if we are easily influenced by others' arguments and desires?

A second way that the excessive uptaker might be seen to develop a bad character trait over time is when she is so committed to giving others uptake that she puts off decision-making. Thinking that she must hear everyone out before taking action, she judiciously weighs each speaker evenly and fairly and avoids the rush-to-judgment, unfortunately, too long. Part of getting it right about any virtue is that there is a right time to decide and to act, and the excessive uptaker, in the interest of being inclusive, may miss the moment again and again. Being trustworthy is more than an orientation toward others; it is something that we exhibit in action and feeling. And it means that sometimes we must make choices to come down on one side or another.

8.2.5 Back to the opening example

Let's consider the vignette in 8.1 now, applying an understanding of the virtue of giving uptake. I will call attention to three points in that exchange where uptake is given. First, note that the clinician is prepared to discuss the patient's absence from last week's session and asks for an explanation. After receiving the explanation that the patient had overslept because she'd taken a much-needed sleeping pill, the clinician first empathized with the patient's need for sleep before continuing with the inquiry ('That's a tough spot to be in'). I take the clinician's pause in pursuit of an explanation to be an example of giving uptake because the clinician takes seriously the patient's dilemma and responds to it directly and empathetically. That response tells the patient that, even though she missed an appointment as a result of oversleeping, she is seen by her clinician as a person with a broader life than merely a patient who fills a time slot. Secondly, when the clinician asks the patient how late she slept, the patient (probably rightly) took the question to ascertain whether or not the patient still could have made the appointment and decided not to. The patient responded with irritation, feeling defensive. Here, too, the clinician gave uptake to the irritation even when it was not expressed verbally ('You sound irritated'). This was an important point in the dialogue because it gave the message that it was okay for the patient to be irritated with her therapist, and it opened up a space for the patient to own her irritation. It is especially important in light of the ways in which women's anger, and in particular, BPD patients' anger, is misunderstood, as I argued in Chapter 2. Thirdly, when the patient explained her irritation in terms of feeling accused of not wanting to come to the appointment, the therapist reassures her that the issue is that therapy is valuable, thereby reaching out to the patient without engaging her defensiveness. ('Well, I'm sorry you missed').[1] By acknowledging that the patient faces a genuine dilemma of 'sleep versus therapy appointment,' the clinician indicates to the patient that her problem is taken seriously and needs to be addressed. Note that, at least in this exchange, the clinician isn't digging deeper into possible acting out that the patient might be doing by missing an appointment; the patient's explanation is taken at the face value. This is important in the light of the tendency I've noted for clinicians to attribute negative motives and attitudes too quickly.

8.3 Applications to BPD patients

8.3.1 Giving uptake to patients who self-injure

Let me now fill out these ideas a bit more. Clinicians are often at a loss to understand the actions of individuals who self-injure. Many find it difficult to talk about the self-injury in a way that allows the patient a role as an interpreter of her own signs (Favazza 1996; Himber 1994). 'Ross and McKay (1979) found that only after conceding that they did not understand self-mutilation were counselors then able to suspend clinical judgment and allow the young women to explain their behavior' (Zila and Kiselica 2001). In analyzing the logic of communication, H. P. Grice introduced principles and maxims for conversation such as 'Do not make your contribution more informative than is required,' 'Be relevant,' and 'Do not say that for which you lack adequate evidence' (Grice 1989, pp. 26–27). Extrapolating freely from Grice's maxims, I offer five communicative maxims to guide the giving of uptake where the focus of therapy is self-injurious behavior of people diagnosed with BPD. (In other words, these maxims are for a restricted domain; they may not apply for other diagnoses or for other identifying behaviors of BPD). I then sketch out how these maxims apply to giving uptake to patients' anger.

---

[1] However, the therapist's comment, 'I'm sorry you missed' is not unambiguous; the comment could be interpreted as an evasion of confrontation or even as an indirect criticism of the missed appointment. I think it leans toward reassurance in that the therapist does avoid engaging the patient in confrontation or criticism and, instead, highlights the point that a missed meeting is a professional disappointment to any therapist who is engaged in seeing his or her patient make progress in therapy.

8.3.2 **Five maxims for clinical use**

8.3.2.a Approach discussions of self-injury with the Principle of Charity

The Principle of Charity holds that, rather than thinking that what a person has communicated is false, we try to interpret what a person communicates as true. I suggest that clinicians employ this principle when talking with BPD patients about self-injurious behavior. According to philosopher Donald Davidson, a theory of meaning allows us correctly to interpret the communications of others. But we don't yet have an adequate theory of meaning when it comes to self-injurious behavior, so we cannot know *a priori* what meaning a given self-injurious act has (cf. Miller 1998, pp. 263–273). If understanding a patient involves something like interpretation, then we can either aim for preserving truth in a communicative exchange or for preserving meaning. Davidson's argument is that a theory of meaning ought to adopt the Principle of Charity as an attitude an interpreter takes *before* he or she can interpret.

I recognize the contentiousness of suggesting that patients diagnosed with BPD be approached with the Principle of Charity. Such patients may have cognitive difficulties that hamper their grasp on reality, so readers may question the value of assuming communicator truth in those cases (Gunderson 2001; Kroll 1988). On the other hand, the two main problem areas for BPD patients – reality testing and thought processes – occur mostly under episodes of stress and seem to be relatively strong and intact otherwise (Goldstein 1995). So, let me try to motivate this maxim.

The argument I have advanced concerning self-injury is that it can be located among various body modifications found across cultures. It is unwise to assume *a priori* that we know what a given signification of this sort means. It is important to resist the rush to judgment that a patient's actions are irrational or pathological without exploring the patient's own interpretations and explanations for her behavior. What I am suggesting here, then, is that clinicians should assume that the patient has beliefs which, by our lights, are true (Miller 1998, p. 270). What this amounts to is that the clinician hold beliefs constant as far as possible while solving for meaning (Miller 1998, p. 270). The value in this approach is that it slows down the interpretive process and shifts more of the right and responsibility for meaning-making to the patient. Adopting this principle, then, would create a space for the clinician to interpret *with* her patient the actions under scrutiny, while allowing the patient to take the lead. In giving uptake to patients who self-injure, clinicians are allowing patients to make meaning and to experience themselves as would-be knowers. And clinicians will be exhibiting dispositional features of trustworthiness such as being epistemically responsible and paying attention to the particular patient (see Chapter 7).

Note that this maxim applies to a very restricted domain: it concerns patients diagnosed with BPD, and only with respect to communications about self-injury. What I am proposing, in effect, is that clinicians bracket off their evaluative skills and capacities to the degree that they are not distracted by judgments about the truth value while therapeutic work is being done on the subject of self-injury.

8.3.2.b Take a critical and reflective stance toward your own conceptual framework

While none of us can step outside of culture altogether, we can evaluate our attitudes, beliefs, and values from a second-order level (Taylor 1989, Frankfurt 2005). Complete objectivity is an unlikely ideal. But clinicians can, and should, think critically about ways in which prevailing norms and values may be influencing their understanding of the world and their ways of being in it. They need to be on guard against subtle assumptions about health, rationality, and good actions that could be misguided in the case of a particular patient and thereby inhibit that patient's ability to heal. This maxim probably has more general application and should be kept in a close pocket to remember.

8.3.2.c Adopt a position of epistemic humility and moral uncertainty about meanings and explanations for self-injury

Related to the last maxim, this one encourages the clinician to be open to discovery. In order to do that, the clinician needs to be somewhat skeptical toward her own confidence level with respect to general meanings about self-injury. She should suspend judgment to the degree she is able without jeopardizing short-term physical safety of the patient. Clinicians must be concerned about imminent danger, so this maxim cannot always be applied. But taking a longer range view, this heuristic allows the clinician to work with the patient in exploring meaning and to participate in meaning-making that isn't prematurely closed off. This maxim takes time in order fully to be followed, so the clinician should be aware that it requires persistent vigilance against closure.

8.3.2.d Recognize that the patient, too, may bring assumptions about her behavior that are culturally inflected

This is, perhaps, a call for balance between adopting the Principle of Charity, on the one hand, and taking the patient's point of view as the final one, on the other hand. Taking an explanation or a meaning as true, in this case, does not commit the clinician to any particular theory of truth. Patients may be believed about their own interpretations, but clinicians and patients together may want to unpack patients' conceptual frameworks, regarding self-injury. Patients are likely to pick up the idea that people who self-injure are pathologically demented, and that attitude may be expressed by the patient in therapy, but it is important to try to identify whether the patient is distressed by her own behavior or whether she just believes that she ought to be.

8.3.2.e When asked to give an interpretation, offer disjunctive ones

Sometimes a patient will ask the clinician for assistance in understanding her actions, and sometimes the clinician will want to offer alternative interpretations to the one the patient is offering. In the spirit of openness and a commitment to patient autonomy, clinicians should offer an array of interpretations so that the patient can explore various possibilities to see which best fits. Or, the patient and clinician may brainstorm together about possible meanings. The point is not to impose an interpretation that the clinician thinks is correct, and not to close off opportunities for discovery or new knowledge. When offering disjunctive possibilities for interpretation, the clinician may need to avoid simple either/or statements, as borderline patients are already prone to thinking in dichotomous extremes and need to be encouraged to think in more complex terms.

The aim of these maxims is to preserve the integrity of the communicator vis-à-vis her unfolding understanding of her self-injurious behavior. The value in it is that it facilitates greater understanding of the patient's experience. Let me now briefly address another difficult issue for clinicians who work with BPD patients: patient anger, again applying the idea of uptake and offering maxims.

8.4 Uptake and anger

I argued in Chapter 2 that patient anger intersects with norms for appropriate expressions of anger and, especially, gender norms for anger and that those norms make it difficult for clinicians to respond empathetically to patient anger. I described what I call the doubling effect of anger and urged clinicians to create a space for real-time anger toward them to be addressed. An example of a clinician doing this is found in the opening example, when the clinician picks up on the patient's irritation and says 'You sound irritated.' The clinician doesn't assume that the irritation is merely an echo of how the patient feels about past slights by primary caregivers but, instead, that it is probably due to the clinician's pressing the patient on how long she overslept. I said that this is an example of giving uptake.

The maxims offered for giving uptake to patients' self-injurious behavior are useful here, too, but need to be unpacked differently with respect to anger. The Principle of Charity would seem to require clinicians to assume that the patient has a reason to be angry in the here and now. That is, the clinician would approach the patient as reasonable and her anger as *prima facie* warranted. This principle applies to two aspects of patient anger: that her anger is *prima facie* warranted and that she should be the primary meaning-maker of her anger. This principle should be considered even when the patient is not very good at expressing her anger. For example, she may raise her voice, or cry, or stomp out of a session, and then return sullenly. Rachel Reiland (2004) reports her sometimes vicious name-calling at her clinician, Dr. Padgett. The Principle of Charity calls for clinicians to be fairly open to a range of expressions of anger so as not automatically to pathologize it (cf. Chapter 2). This may mean that the clinician stay relatively detached about the name-calling directed at her, while at the same time being empathetic to the anger itself.

But sometimes, a patient who is told to do something she doesn't want to do will become violent and threatening and will need to be put in restraints. This is not the time to practice the Principle of Charity – we must act. This is why it is important to situate giving uptake as a virtue: it has a mean and extremes. We can give uptake too broadly, too much for a given situation, as in a patient who is violent. The Doctrine of the Mean reminds us that virtue is found 'at the right time, in the right way, toward the right end,' and so on (Aristotle 1985).

The second maxim that clinicians should take a critical and reflective stance toward their own conceptual frameworks and values also applies. As a general maxim, it is probably second nature to many clinicians. But when it comes to BPD anger (or manipulativity, say), clinicians may have prejudices and blind spots, and their training and experience may reinforce cultural biases. Clinicians will be in a better position to give uptake properly when they have examined the extent to which their beliefs about women's anger affects their ability to take angry women seriously and to correct false assumptions.

Epistemic humility, the third maxim to apply to the virtue of giving uptake, is connected to the second maxim and also to the moral requirement that we take our epistemic responsibilities seriously, a point argued in Chapter 7. Understanding BPD patients' anger is especially difficult; it has a doubling effect, which is challenging to unravel while at the same time giving uptake when appropriate; it is cast as pathological too quickly in clinical settings; it is saturated with moral value that is gendered; and it is sometimes genuinely frightening and dangerous. It is important to appreciate the complexity of BPD anger in order properly to address it when the patient communicates this anger.

As with self-injury, anger is culturally inflected and patients also bring in their cultural assumptions and beliefs about it. A prevalent attitude about a woman's anger is that she is a bitch, and a patient may believe that about herself. Anger may be an especially difficult issue for women who come from cultures where they are expected to be subservient and passive; these women may feel deeply ashamed and afraid of their feelings of anger, let alone the expression of it. In order to give uptake properly to a patient who believes her anger is usually inappropriate, extreme, or proof that she is bad, morally flawed, or mentally unstable, the clinician needs to help the patient dispel such beliefs.

Finally, when asked to give an interpretation, offer disjunctive ones. Most clinicians are trained to do this and so this maxim is not new. But it bears repeating in its application to anger in BPD patients. We have seen that these patients' anger can be big and rageful, frightening and intimidating; but it can also collide with cultural norms for women's expression of anger and be interpreted in a distorted manner. Since the aim of the virtue of giving uptake is to facilitate communication that preserves the integrity of the communicator, it is important not to 'tell' the patient what her anger means or what has prompted her anger. Again, clinicians know this – but sometimes they move toward closure of an interpretation in an unconscious effort to control a climate that feels chaotic (perhaps to the patient as well as the clinician). For this reason, I emphasize this well-known maxim. And, in light of the previous maxim – that clinicians need to consider the beliefs and assumptions that the patient brings to the therapeutic relationship – disjunctive interpretations should aim to open up a space where culturally shameful anger, or anger as a bad character trait in women, holds the possibility of transforming into acceptable anger.

8.5 Conclusion

The last section illustrates a heuristic that clinicians can follow when cultivating the virtue of giving uptake rightly. These maxims are rules of thumb, not principles or hard-and-fast guidelines. Keep in mind that giving uptake to patients need not assume that patients are irrational or unable to be reasonable in some domains and some settings. But neither does it mean that, when patients are irrational or when their mental disorder gets in the way of communicating or being understood, clinicians do not need to give uptake to their patients.

Giving uptake is a difficult virtue to learn. I speculate that the reason is that, unlike trustworthiness or empathy, uptake in general is an unknown concept for most people and especially when it is called a virtue. It doesn't have the familiarity of other long-standing moral practices such as being trustworthy or being empathetic. While the skill of being a good listener has currency, it only captures the more superficial aspect of giving uptake. Giving uptake involves not only the moral and epistemic qualities of attentiveness and world-traveling, but also the political potential of claim-making and rights recognition. To do all of this with another is to draw upon a rich background of understanding about the world of structural inequalities, silence and voice, authority and subjugation, and suffering and healing. The virtue of giving uptake needs to be cultivated in us and to become practice, but since it is new as a moral and epistemic concept, it also needs to be theorized and expanded upon.

Despite the difficulty of learning the landscape of giving uptake – or perhaps because of it – clinicians must engage in practical reasoning and development of a critical consciousness in order to find the mean in giving uptake. And again, they will need to have other virtues as well as other moral and epistemic abilities, such as world-traveling, attentiveness, and empathy. It is to this last concept that I now turn.

Chapter 9

Situating empathy in our lives

9.1 **Introduction**

As we have seen throughout this book, the absence of empathy toward BPD patients is anathema to successful therapeutic relations and patients' potential healing. This last chapter on virtues, therefore, focuses on the importance of cultivating clinician empathy. I begin this chapter with a discussion of how a deficiency in empathy toward these patients raises difficult questions about the status of BPD as a personality disorder. Thus, this chapter brings together questions of empathy and blame, disorder and responsibility that resonate throughout much of the book. I have placed this discussion at the end of the book instead of at the beginning because I believe readers are now in a better position to think critically about the status of BPD as a personality disorder. Keep in mind, though, that I am not arguing that it is not a PD but that careful analytic and scientific work lies ahead of us in order to answer the many questions that this book raises. I am arguing that, to the extent that the symptoms of BPD are picking out a genuine disorder, they ought to be met with the empathy appropriate to the suffering and distress that anyone living with mental illness experiences. I argue that an understanding of a particular kind of empathy, called controlled empathy, is crucial for clinicians to develop in order for them to work with BPD patients.

9.2 **What's at stake**

Evidence abounds that health care workers become alienated from disliked patients, and the effects on patients can be drastic. Clinician negativity toward BPD patients is often self-confirming and self-fulfilling (Bowers 2002, p. 119). Morgan and Priest (1984, 1991) introduced a concept called 'malignant alienation' to call attention to the seriousness of negative interactions between patients and their caregivers. Malignant alienation is a process in which carers become critical of patients who they perceive as provocative and unreasonable, and the effects on those patients are, literally, lethal.

Morgan and Priest found that a significant number of suicides had occurred a short time after patients had become alienated to some degree from others. Bowers, too, found that increased dysfunction and suicidal behavior are correlated with negative reactions by staff (Bowers 2002, p. 18). Negative views of BPD patients can be used against them in legal cases, too: in a disciplinary hearing in Toronto in 2004 of a physician for alleged sexual abuse of his BPD patient, the defense lawyer argued not that sexual activities did not occur but that the woman was 'a calculated manipulator and liar' (Levy 2004). With the explicit message to jurors that the patient was not to be trusted, jurors were unlikely to believe the patient's allegations that she was abused and, thus, were unlikely to be sympathetic to claims that she was traumatized and damaged. The courts thereby may re-victimize a patient, compounding any damage that may have been done initially. The point is that patients are not likely to get better without experiencing empathetic responses from clinicians and others.

9.2.1 Willful madness or, Morality and mental illness reprise (from 6.6)

That BPD patients *do* evoke negative responses is unquestionable – but the reasons are more complex than that patients just *are* particularly difficult. As Mary Zanarini says, '[p]eople don't burn "I'm a bad person" into their arm with a cigarette because they are difficult' (McIlroy 2004); the Diagnostic and Statistical Manual (DSM) and International Classification of Diseases (ICD) classifications hold that people with BPD have a serious illness. But an examination of actual practice suggests that many clinicians and carers don't quite believe that. For example, in one report, the authors describe the patient's behavior as deliberate: 'Her pain medication was administered through a patient-controlled analgesic pump; her use of these medications appeared selective, increasing markedly when her husband or therapists were in the room' (Harvey and Watters 1998, p. 122). The patient is reported as angrily refusing psychiatric involvement; behaving in resistant and non-compliant ways; and behaving in ways that frustrated and demoralized staff (p. 122). The authors suggest that '[i]t may be helpful to view this behavior as a *strategy that borderline patients use…*' (Harvey and Watters 1998, p. 124; emphasis added).

Research by Bowers found that psychiatric nurses were 'virtually unanimous that PD patients are responsible either completely or to some degree' (Bowers 2002, p. 84). They reason that, unless a patient is deluded or hallucinating, or confused or muddled, she knows what she is doing and is therefore responsible for what she does (Bowers 2002, p. 85). And Theodore Millon's language and use of scare quotes suggests that he, too, views BPD behavior as deliberate.

> Depression serves as an instrument for them to frustrate and retaliate against those who have 'failed' them or 'demanded too much.' Angered by the 'inconsiderateness' of others, these borderlines employ their somber and melancholy sadness as a vehicle to get back at

them or teach them a lesson. Moreover, by exaggerating their plight and by moping about helplessly, they effectively avoid responsibilities, place added burdens on others, and thereby cause their families not only to take care of them but to suffer and feel guilt while doing so. In addition, the dour moods and excessive complaints of these border-lines infect the atmosphere with tension and irritability, thereby upsetting what equa-nimity remains among those who have 'disappointed' them.

(Millon 1996, p. 663)

In fact, Millon's account almost suggests that borderline patients are scamming their illness in order to manipulate others.

The idea that BPD patients are being calculatingly difficult is, as we saw in Chapter 6, widely held. And linked with that view is the reasoning that, since they're behaving badly on purpose, they are responsible for their behavior and therefore are to blame for it. They aren't mad after all – they're just bad.

Theory and practice are at odds here, and I point out the consequences of this apparent inconsistency.

Can you blame someone and still be empathetic with them? Apparently not – when it comes to patients diagnosed with BPD. In one study, researchers set out to answer the question: Do patients diagnosed with BPD receive qualitatively different care from patients diagnosed with other [non-personality-disordered] diagnoses? Hypothetical vignettes in which the only variable was the presence or absence of a diagnosis of BPD suggested that stereotyped perceptions play a cru-cial role in how the behavior of BPD patients is interpreted and responded to. 'The difficult behavior of the patient with borderline personality disorder is often seen as "bad" and "deliberate" rather than as "sick"…The schizophrenic patient, on the other hand, is not perceived as having this control' (Gallop *et al.* 1989, p. 815). Schizophrenic patients are perceived as ill, whereas 'borderline patients… do not meet the criteria of "good and attractive" patients. They are not perceived as sick, compliant, cooperative, or grateful' (Gallop *et al.* 1989, p. 819).

In terms of quality of care, nurses were more likely to give responses that were belittling or contradicting if the patient's diagnosis was BPD and were likely to be empathetic toward schizophrenics. The researchers conclude that 'the label [BPD] is sufficient to diminish staff's expressed empathy…' (Gallop *et al.* 1989, p. 815). Clinicians and staff seem to believe that BPD patients 'deserve' less empathetic treatment and that their diagnosis means that they are 'bad' or manipulative (Gallop *et al.* 1989, p. 818; Bowers 2002).

To flesh out the issue of responsibility and blame, I turn to what is called 'attribu-tion theory.' This theory is based on the idea that people infer (i.e. attribute) causes for events in order to gain a sense of control over their environment (Markham and Trower 2003, p. 245). When we attribute control to another person for causing a negative event, we are more likely to react negatively to them. 'An example [of Weiner's model (1985)] might be illustrated by considering our responses to a negative event, such as a car traveling very slowly in front of us on the road. If we make the attribution that the driver is *choosing* to go slowly (has control), [Weiner's] [attribution] theory would suggest that we are likely to experience anger' (Markham and Trower 2003, p. 245.)

Using this theory, researchers in several studies have found that, when clinicians and carers attribute to a patient the ability to control her behavior, they experience more anger and less empathy (cf. Sharrock *et al.* 1990; Dagnan *et al.* 1998; Bowers 2002). For example, in Markham and Trower's 2003 study, staff were told to consider a patient with one of three diagnoses: BPD, schizophrenia, or depression. They were then presented with six short scenarios of challenging behaviors of patients such as violent behavior, setting off a fire alarm, not attending a meeting, refusing to carry out a request by staff. They were asked to generate one central cause for each of the behaviors. They were also asked to rate their sympathy with the patient in each scenario. This study, like previous ones, found that staff were much more likely to attribute control of the cause of negative events for patients diagnosed with BPD than either schizophrenia or depression. It also found that the mean sympathy ratings for BPD patients fell toward 'unsympathetic' whereas the mean sympathy ratings for schizophrenic or depressed patients fell toward 'extremely sympathetic' (Markham and Trowers 2003, p. 251). Another study found that clinicians who perceived themselves as being manipulated by their patients feel strongly negative toward those patients (Bowers 2003, p. 329). Furthermore, as we saw in Chapter 6, evidence shows that clinicians and carers who work with BPD patients come to clinic with a ready-made scheme of interpretation that shapes their perception (Bowers 2003, p. 327). For example, Bowers argues that the idea of the 'manipulative borderline' is so entrenched that clinicians *a priori* assume these patients act on manipulative motives, and then perceive what they already expected to see (Bowers 2003, p. 327).

To summarize the argument so far: a central aspect of clinicians' feelings of anger and entrapment toward BPD patients is the attribution of choice and responsibility to the patient. Studies have found that clinicians tend to impute the ability to have self-control to BPD patients in comparison with other diagnoses and, then, blame them for their behavior. With a template in place that encourages interpretations of behavior negatively, clinicians are less likely to be empathetic. A patient may be difficult at the outset, but she may also be 'difficult' in response to the reception she is getting. This is a dynamic rooted in interpretation that is partly diagnosis-driven, and it looks like we are confronting a nasty form of loopiness (Hacking 1999, pp. 105 and 121). This idea needs some expanding.

Ian Hacking introduced what he calls 'the looping effect of human kinds' (1999, p. 34), kinds that are contrasted with 'indifferent' ones. The latter are things like quarks and microbes that, although they interact with humans, are not aware of human classifications of them as quarks and microbes. Being aware of how we are categorized, stereotyped – or, for our purposes, diagnosed – can lead us to us experience ourselves differently and even change our behavior, emotions, attitudes, and beliefs in response to that awareness (Hacking 1999, p. 105). Hacking does not reject the possibility that some neuropathology that is an indifferent kind might explain a mental disorder; his point is that the *idea* of a particular psychopathology and the *people* diagnosed with that psychopathology do indeed interact and change human behavior. It is this dynamic that is of interest to me with respect to BPD. The reason I claim that the looping effect between the diagnosis BPD and those who carry that diagnosis is nasty is that it can do so much damage to the patients that clinicians are trying to serve. Furthermore, the loopiness, in this case, twists and distorts BPD to such a degree that the status of the diagnosis is called into question.

9.2.2 What is a personality disorder, and why does the answer matter?

I'll start with the question, Why are BPD patients so disliked? Is it true that they are PIAs (pains in the ass, cf. Chapter 6)? Let's look at an example:

> Therapy with Ms. C seemed off to an uneventful start, that is, until the fifth week. In the first session, I had told Ms. C that my usual policy was to charge for missed sessions, unless I could fill the time. I had said that I would be willing to discuss this matter if she had any misgivings about it, with the clear implication that there was flexibility. When Ms. C offered no objections, we moved on. Then in the fifth week, Ms. C said she had been thinking about my fee policy, in fact had become increasingly obsessed about it. Her conclusion was that it was totally unacceptable. After considerable discussion I said that although I had originally felt that the policy was reasonable, I could understand her objections, and because of those, the policy would not apply to her. This, however, did not eliminate the issue. The fee policy became the main topic, session after session. Ms C expressed her opinion that even though the fee policy would not apply to her, it was clear evidence that I was insensitive, unconcerned, inclined to treat her unfairly, and only interested in money. She thought it would be difficult to work with such a self-centered, unempathetic, and money-oriented individual. As other evidence of my lack of concern and insensitivity entered into the hours, such as my letting her in a minute late on one occasion, my taking a week's vacation, my diverting my attention from her by turning on the air conditioner, and my occasionally moving about in a restless way, Ms. C concluded that it would be absolutely useless to continue treatment with me. After exploration of these issues I referred her to a colleague.

> (Goldstein 1995)

Ms C *does* sound like a difficult patient; it is not surprising that her onslaught of criticism and accusation would evoke negative emotions. The question I want to focus on from this example is whether or not Ms C is being deliberately difficult and, so, blameworthy. Viewing her as such is consistent with most attitudes toward BPD patients. Is it appropriate to hold her accountable, disliking her for being relentlessly critical and accusatory? Bowers writes that:

> The generally hopeless, pessimistic, angry attitudes of carers can be seen to originate in the difficult behaviours of PD patients. They bully, con, capitalize, divide, condition, and corrupt those around them. They make complaints over inconsequential or non-existent issues in order to manipulate the staff. They can be seriously violent over unpredictable and objectively trivial events, or may harm and disfigure themselves in ways that have an intense emotional impact on staff. If this were not enough, they also behave in the same way towards each other, provoking serious problems that the staff have to manage and contain.

(Bowers 2002, p. 65)

Bowers certainly captures the way that clinicians perceive and experience BPD patients: patients do morally wrong things like con and corrupt, they do so deliberately, and others' negative responses to them are the fault of the patients. My aim here is not to repudiate the ubiquitous claims about the horrors of working with BPD patients, but to show how conceptual frameworks and perceptions interact with patients to create a destructive dynamic.

We have seen that an assumption prevails that the behaviors of those with BPD are *blameworthy*, and that this amounts to the idea that BPD patients are 'willfully mad.' Let's map out the conceptual terrain.

A personality disorder is said to be 'an enduring pattern of inner experience and behaviour that deviates markedly from the expectations of the individual's culture, is pervasive and inflexible, has an onset in adolescence or early adulthood, is stable over time, and leads to distress or impairment' (DSM-IV-TR 2000, p. 685). The BPD is viewed as an advanced form of structurally defective personality organization, with a moderate-to-severe level of dysfunction (Millon 1996, p. 646).

The question posed in 9.2.2. of this chapter is whether the dysfunctional states, beliefs, desires, and behaviors of BPD are ones that the patient has control over and, if so, which ones. It is crucial to determine this for three reasons: (1) as noted earlier, moral philosophy holds that people ought not to be blamed for things that are beyond their control; (2) mistakes in holding BPD patients responsible impede treatment and may make patients worse. On the other hand, (3) if patients are pretty much in control of their beliefs, desires, and behaviors, it's not clear that they have a dysfunction that fits PD theory. I'll set out the issues that require clarification in order to make epistemically responsible judgments about responsibility and blame regarding these patients.

Amanda Bray sets out two fairly standard conditions for the correct functioning of decision-making faculty and therefore for responsible action: (1) that the person knows the facts that are needed to make the correct action in a given situation. This requires accurate perception, the ability to distinguish relevant from irrelevant facts, and the ability to learn facts and, (2) that the person makes rational causal inferences between different mental representations concerning the action (Bray 2003, p. 272). Bray's account is consistent with my discussion of deliberation in Chapter 4: in order to be responsible for one's actions, one needs to have chosen freely – meaning without force or coercion. When a person is forced to do something, she cannot have done otherwise. If she cannot have done otherwise, she cannot be said to have chosen, and therefore cannot be held responsible (for that action). Coercion is the explanans[1] when the choices available to one are arranged or structured such that the most attractive choice to the agent is one that the agent would not choose if things weren't structured this way. The agent is still making a choice, but (in this domain) her choice is internally coerced. Controversy exists about whether or not to hold people accountable for coerced actions. Existentialists hold us responsible on the grounds that there is always an alternative action to be taken (namely, death; cf. Sartre 2003), whereas Aristotle says that almost no coerced actions are blameworthy (Aristotle NE 1999; Bk iii). The latter view sees coercion as a matter of degree. So, for instance, if a robber holds a gun to your head and says 'Your money or your life,' you are likely to give the robber your money. This is direct coercion. But women might claim to be coerced into avoiding bars at night, or going on walks in the woods alone, and this kind of coercion, although more pervasive, is more subtle.

Chapter 4, on impulsivity, sets out the central questions about responsibility and willing versus having irresistible desires that might mitigate responsibility. We might think of BPD patients as having a volitional disorder, where the problem is in terms of the structure of the will. Freedom and responsibility, on this view, require not only being able to choose between available alternatives, but also to be able to choose which desires one wants to *have* – in other words, in order to say one has deliberately chosen her action, it must be the case that the person has control of the structure of her will (Frankfurt 2005). Harry Frankfurt's account of freedom and responsibility – as a matter of whether the desires we have are the ones we want to have – better captures the struggle most

---

[1] The explanans is a term from philosophy of science that refers to the explanatory premises; its associated term is the explanandum, which refers to the thing that needs explaining.

self-harming patients experience than merely as a battle between competing desires. A case in point: one patient I talked with, who repeatedly seriously harms herself, says she doesn't want to feel this way – she doesn't want to have the desire to cut herself. In other words, at a second-order level, she wants not to want what she, at the first-order level, wants. But she believes she has no control over the structure of her will – that her second-order desires are unable to govern her will.

Are patients who engage in SIB or have hard-to-resist impulses to blame for their actions? The answer partly depends on how they came by their desires and distresses, matters currently being researched by developmental psychiatrists and brain scientists. If BPD patients are unable to structure their will such that their second-order desires take primacy in decision-making and action, then responsibility for their dysfunctional behavior is at least mitigated. It also depends on whether one can be compelled to action and yet approach that action calculatively. As many carers view BPD patients as calculative, they take such behaviors to be evidence that they were not compelled.

Now of course, just because someone is mentally ill, it doesn't mean that every action that person does is out of her control; being mentally ill affects mental faculties relatively, not absolutely (Wilson and Adshead, referring to Buchanan 2004, p. 306.) Furthermore, 'mental faculties affect one *another* and are interconnected' (Wilson and Adshead referring to Buchanan 2004, p. 306). While some mental state changes may be under conscious control, others may not be (Wilson and Adshead 2004, p. 306).

Let's return to the example of the 'difficult' patient, Ms. C. Does her personality disorder exculpate her from blame for her critical and demanding attitude toward the clinician? Presumably, that she may not perceive him or their interactions accurately is a result of her disorder. That she interprets him wrongly is also an effect of the disorder. That she is making unreasonable demands is said to be a characteristic of the disorder. Action by action, we might say she could have done otherwise, but if we view BPD as a mental disorder, the cluster of symptoms makes it less plausible to hold the patient responsible for expressing her disorder through her behavior. Is she able to recognize and correct mistaken judgments in perception and interpretation of her therapist? Is she able to be in control of her anger and hostility?

If we want to preserve the BPD construct as some kind of disorder, a central part of the task will be to get much clearer on what kinds of mental faculties are affected and how they are affected. We need to know 'how much of what kind' and to what degree they affect a patient's agency. It will not do for clinicians simply to make assumptions about freedom and responsibility when it comes to these patients. Zanarini *et al.* (1998) found that 'some borderline patients reported suffering for high percentages of the time for reasons and in ways that nonborderline patients rarely do…The intensity of pain and the amount of time suffering pain reported by borderline patients proves, by itself, easily capable of discriminating patients with BPD from those without' (quoted from Gunderson 2001, p. 13). As John Gunderson puts it, 'it is a terrible way to experience life' (Gunderson 2001, p. 13). If BPD is a genuine disorder, patients who suffer from it deserve empathy, not blame.

But it looks like many clinicians and carers do hold a view of BPD patients as morally flawed and choosing to be that way. So, I return to the question of why these patients are so readily blamed when other mentally ill patients are excused. I identify three values that I think are embedded in responses to these patients.

1. They're needy and clinging when the measure of psychological maturity is autonomy. Dependence and neediness are scorned in medical and popular domains alike. Desperation exposes extreme vulnerability, and BPD patients often are desperate to avoid abandonment. People in western cultures don't like to be face to face with desperation: we are uncomfortable with vulnerability and weakness.

2. They do things that make others feel grossed out and disgusted, like slashing open their arms or burning their thighs. Disgust is a moral emotion, and when it is evoked by the actions of another person, the person feeling disgust is likely to blame that person for causing the disgust.

3. Zanarini remarks that borderline patients 'are not as docile and respectful as other patients' (McIlroy 2004). Noncompliant and disrespectful behavior is negatively valued in itself, but it also intersects with gender values in most cultures. Femininity carries with it ideas of submissiveness rather than aggression, and respect and nurturance toward others rather than demandingness and entitlement toward self. It's important to view BPD in the light of social values about gender: women are far more likely to be diagnosed with BPD than are men (Jimenez 1997; APA 2001). As noted in the Introduction, the picture of the borderline patient as a manipulative, demanding, aggressive, and angry woman is a recurring theme over the past 20 years.

These values are mixed in with confusion about the extent to which BPD patients *are* responsible for their dysfunctional behavior. Taken together, clinicians' conceptual frameworks and perceptions put treatment at risk: blaming, negative, and rejecting attitudes in clinicians impede their ability to be empathetic.

9.3 **Empathy as a concept, empathy as a virtue**

In the following sections, I start from a theoretical framework. First, I set out a philosophical definition of empathy and explain empathy's role in social relations. Then, I situate empathy as a virtue, with extremes and a mean. In 9.4., I apply the virtue of empathy to the practice of therapeutic work with BPD patients.

9.3.1 **The concept**

Part of being a moral person is the recognition that our actions, choices, and ways of being in the world affect others in ways sometimes insignificant, sometimes profound, and that this recognition of relationship matters to us. Moral frameworks, especially those systematized in philosophical theories, function as guidelines for impartial, rational, and moral decision-making. But as I discussed in Chapter 3, a conception of the good moral agent that valorizes the autonomous man who is self-sufficient, rational, and impartial paints an impoverished picture of the moral landscape and of human psychology, and recent moral philosophy has attended carefully to the flaws in mainstream theories. Critics argue for (and I enthusiastically endorse) a more realistic and complete picture of morality where humans are conceptualized as relational and as working to honor our emotional, cognitive, and material connections as constituents of the moral life.

Still, this relational quality of morality is sometimes painfully difficult to put into practice, and not only in the psychiatric domain. As William Ickes writes in the introduction to *Empathic Accuracy:*

> ...the indeterminate, ever-elusive nature of the Other's subjective experience when the Other is immanently present is a central problem not just for phenomenologists and existential philosophers. It is a central problem for all of us. When the strange figure abruptly looms on Ortega [y Gasset's] horizon, or slips past the park benches to disorder [Jean-Paul] Sartre's private world, he reminds us all how difficult — and yet how important — it is to accurately infer the thoughts, feelings, motives, and intentions of other people.

> (Ickes 1997, p.1)

If we want to create better moral relations – more peaceful, more just, richer in vitality, and flourishing for all – it is imperative that we understand moral psychology in all its complexity and messiness.

Empathic emotions are central to recognizing the subjectivity and humanity of others:

> Emotions anchor us to the particular moral circumstance, to the aspect of a situation that addresses us immediately, to the here and now. To "see" the circumstance and

to see oneself as addressed by it, and thus to be susceptible to the way a situation affects the weal and woe of others, in short, to identify a situation as carrying moral significance in the first place — all of this is required in order to enter the domain of the moral, and none of it would come about without the basic emotional faculty of empathy.

(Vetlesen 1994, p. 4)

Empathy is a kind of moral perception that involves attentiveness and place-taking — which, Vetlesen notes, requires both that we see and that we listen (I would say, give uptake rightly). Iris Murdoch also emphasizes the moral effort required to be attentive, pointing out that being good is not merely a matter of discrete right actions but of the moral vision we cultivate in between the moments of choosing: 'I can only choose within the world I can see, in the moral sense of "see" which implies that clear vision is a result of moral imagination and moral effort' (Murdoch 1970, p. 37).

Sara Hodges and Daniel Wegner capture the depth of the task we face in being empathic for even one specific encounter:

> To empathize with a person in a situation involves more than simply changing one's spatial viewpoint; it also involves changing one's judgment of the situation, one's memory for events and one's emotional responsiveness to them, one's conception of the person's traits and goals, and even one's conception of oneself.... The occurrence of empathy involves such a generalized structural transformation in thought and emotion that it must be conceptualized more broadly than many less sweeping changes in mental content.

(Hodges and Wegner 1997, p. 312)

Hodges and Wegner make a crucial point for my purposes. Clinicians and carers who work with BPD patients need to have a rich concept of empathy that they also know how to employ. The clinical literature that mentions the term but doesn't unpack it is not helpful. Furthermore, it isn't enough merely to know intellectually what empathy is; paraphrasing Aristotle, I remind readers that our aim in ethical inquiry is not to know what empathy is but to know how to become empathetic. Virtues, such as empathy, are to be expressed in order to facilitate genuine flourishing, or at least a degree of healing through connection, mutual trust, and other moral attributes.

I take empathy to be a vitally important character trait not only for individual flourishing but also for social harmony and morally good relationships. As Arne Vetlesen says, 'In moral performance a great deal turns on whether the other is perceived as an abstract, faceless, and "formal" other or as a concrete other to which I can relate emotionally as well as intellectually' (Vetlesen 1994, p. 287). Empathy is a rich moral and epistemological concept, the cultivation of which is critical to good therapy.

9.3.2 **The virtue of empathy**

Empathy is not only a central moral concept; it is a virtue . In saying that it is a virtue, I mean that it contributes to flourishing, it has a mean and extremes, and it is voluntary. In the last chapter, we considered what the world would be like if we did not have rights (Joel Feinberg's 'Nowheresville') and determined that the ability to make claims is central to living with dignity and voice. We similarly might consider what the world would be like without empathy. With respect to trust, we come to know the value of others' trustworthiness in part by the recognition that we cannot always take care of the things we value by ourselves and so, sometimes, need to put our trust in others. This human need also relates to empathy. We all suffer disappointments, fears, anguish, pain, humiliation, and so on. Without empathy, we may suffer alone, a condition that frequently compounds initial suffering. Empathy helps us feel understood and valued in our distress, and this connection itself (cf. Chapter 3 on connection) is sometimes enough partially to relieve that distress. More than that, accurate empathy moves others to action in ways that can help the sufferer. When our daughter Kathy empathized with her aging grandmother's dwindling independence, she came to understand that moving her grandmother out of her home, one of the last bastions of freedom her grandmother has, would break her spirit. Her empathetic attitude and emerging understanding did not come about by her grandmother's remarks but, instead, by Kathy's attentiveness, imaginative place-taking, and deep concern and love for her grandmother's failing health. Kathy conveyed this understanding to us, thereby altering our beliefs about what might be best for this grandmother. Empathy thereby brought about a minimal extension of past flourishing to an elderly widow whose independence is rapidly diminishing. This is a personal and family example, but we should also consider the role that empathy plays in addressing social and health inequalities globally. The poor economy of Haiti, or the human rights violations in the Sudan, or the displaced populations in the Palestinian territories, produce and entrench misery that most of us reading this sort of book will never experience. Many people consider that living under such miserable conditions to be a human rights violation. But as readers will recall from Chapter 8, making a claim against others that a human right has been violated requires that those others give uptake to those claims (not necessarily to agree, though). It may be that empathetic groups and organizations will need to do some footwork before the process of claim-making and giving uptake can occur. Empathy for the misery of others sometimes is all the more affluent and fortunate can offer. But, as with the example of Kathy and her grandmother, empathy can lead to action – which is what I hope would result from empathizing with the suffering majority.

The point of the discussion here is that empathizing with others contributes to their flourishing. But having empathy also contributes to our own flourishing. It draws us out of ourselves; it affirms our humanness by feeling connected to others; it widens our view of the world and the experiences of people; and it increases our self-love. About the latter: Aristotle argued that being a virtuous person requires but also expands self-love (Aristotle 1999, Bk. IX, Ch. 4). Self-love is not to be confused with selfishness; it is a positive and, indeed, necessary quality to possess: friendship is built upon self-love. Aristotle's insight is that the capacity for loving others comes from a sense of worth (virtue, he would say) in ourselves. A virtue like empathy, when exercised, affirms our goodness and worth in that it reminds us that we are capable of morally and epistemically caring about and for others and being moved to alleviate their suffering when able.

The domain of empathy is something like 'feeling-with others and morally attentive place-taking of others.' Like other virtues, empathy has a mean and extremes. The mean concerns feeling-with when appropriate, to the right degree, and for the right (i.e. morally good) reasons (cf. Aristotle 1999, 1106b16–1106b25). What counts as the 'appropriate' and so on is identified by practical reasoning (cf. Chapter 4 on reasoning.) Looking at moral reasoning from an Aristotelian framework, one problem most of us face is in finding the mean between the two extremes of being excessively empathetic (for example, by carrying the emotional burden for others or losing oneself in others) or being deficient in empathy (for example, by consistently failing to be moved by the troubles of others or being unable emotionally and cognitively to imagine others' suffering). The excess is a vice because, among other things, it hampers our own flourishing, and the deficiency is a vice because, among other things, it fails to contribute to the flourishing of others. The clearest way of understanding prevailing attitudes toward BPD patients is, in my view, that some clinicians are deficient in empathy. That is, lack of empathy is not merely a mistake – an action done out of character – but rather is indicative of a settled character flaw – because BPD patients, if they are genuinely personality disordered and thus mentally ill, deserve empathy and not blame, rejection, and dislike.

Although Aristotle did not consider empathy as a virtue, we can plausibly think of empathy as one of the dispositional traits that is necessary to living a good life. First, according to Aristotle, morality is a matter both of feelings and actions; being a morally good person is not merely a matter of reasoning well to right actions – although it is partly that – it also involves 'having the right feelings in the right ways, at the right times, about the right things, towards the right people, for the right end, and in the right way' (Aristotle 1999, 1106b16–1106b25). If clinicians are going to engage with their patients genuinely, they need not only to know intellectually what sorts of attitudes are helpful, but also to learn to have appropriate feelings for their BPD patients. This point seems to be correct in that being moral requires not only that we recognize that what we do and the sorts of persons we are affect others but also that we care about those effects.

Aristotle distinguishes between having a virtue and developing a virtue. Virtue is dispositional, and taking empathy as a virtue, we would say that one who is empathic is the sort of person who has a tendency to feel and act in ways that express care for the perspective and situation of another, finding the intermediate condition. But first we have to practice empathy, developing habits of perception, attitude, inference, and so on, that may not yet express a settled character. Empathy is epistemologically significant in that it allows us to explain and predict the behavior of others, and it is morally significant to our ability appropriately to be responsive/responsible. As Robert Gordon says, 'That is a heavy load for one mental procedure to bear' (Gordon 1995, p. 740).

Virtues are praiseworthy because they are voluntary and up to us (to use Aristotle's language). If they weren't voluntary, we would not praise their expression. Since virtues are said to contribute to living a good (i.e., flourishing) life, it is important to determine whether or not each contender really is under our control. I see empathy as a virtue because empirical evidence suggests that at least one kind of empathy – controlled empathy – is under our control.

In treating empathy as a virtue, I take the position that empathetic responses are, at least to some degree, under our control. But to what extent is the view warranted that empathy can be modulated and controlled? To address this question, let us look more closely at the clinical concept of empathy.

Some researchers suggest that empathy is best thought of as a set of constructs. In particular, that set includes

(a) physiological responses of awareness and arousal;

(b) wandering imagination: a tendency to fantasize and daydream about fictional situations in an undirected manner;

(c) fictional involvement: the ability to transpose oneself by imagination into the feelings and actions of fictitious characters in books, movies, and plays;

(d) humanistic orientation: a sensitivity to and appreciation for the emotional welfare of others; and

(e) emotional contagion: a susceptibility to the emotions of those around one. (Tamborini et al. 1990)

According to these researchers, empathetic processes are understood to involve the somewhat deliberate and conscious place-taking of another and thus are or can be under our control even though awareness and arousal are immediate responses to external stimuli. Reactions are considered empathetic when they are concordant with the observed or likely experience of another and exclude reactions that are discordant. When viewing a horror film, for example, subjects would experience distress and arousal while simultaneously appraising their reactions in terms of concordance or discordance with the victim. When viewers assess their actions as appropriate to the situation that the victim is in, they generate the appropriate emotion by imagining similar situations in their own lives that have produced intense emotional reactions. While this research suggests that there is a cognitive component to empathic responses, it also shows that 'individual differences on various dimensions of empathy have been shown to influence emotional reactions in several distressing contexts' (Tamborini *et al.* 1990, p. 616). Place-taking of another, for example, can occur without an emotional component. Even con artists can engage in place-taking but it then is purely instrumental to the place-taker. Place-taking in itself is not necessarily empathetic; empathy is a reaching out toward another for the other's sake, not one's own.

Other research suggests that some empathic responses (especially in infants) are purely noncognitive in that they do not require recognition of someone else's mental state or a mechanism for converting cognitions into what they are cognitions of. The most basic level of empathic mapping occurs in facial mimicry. Another basic level of empathic mapping is found in social referencing, where the infant refers to the emotional reaction of its primary caregiver to form its own affective appraisal of a novel situation. Social referencing is thought to mark an advance in empathic development in that it involves making inferences from the emotional response of the caregiver to an appropriate response to a new object, although that advance is not yet established empirically. Nevertheless, facial mimicry together with this other level of empathic learning are powerful socializing mechanisms (Gordon 1995, p. 730). What we learn to do, in effect, is to simulate the emotions of others. As Gordon explains, 'simulation permits us to extend to others the modes of attribution, explanation, and prediction that otherwise would be applicable only in our own case' (p. 730). This approach involves a kind of transformation by which one draws an inference from one's own emotion, state of mind, or situational experience (perhaps under a hypothetical situation) to that of another.

> The imaginative shift in the reference of indexicals [from 'I' to 'you' or from 'here' to 'there' or from 'now' to 'then'] reflects a much deeper, more important shift. Many of our tendencies to action or emotion appear to be specially keyed to an egocentric map.
>
> (Gordon 1995, p.734)

So what we can do, through simulation, is to recenter our egocentric map (what Murdoch calls our 'fat relentless ego').

Of course, we have to learn how to make adjustments for errors when simulating the emotions of others because the aim isn't just to simulate others' emotions but to be accurate empathizers.

> Although we imaginatively project ourselves into the person's problem situation, it is always important, in giving advice, to hold back in certain ways from identification with the other person—that is, from making the further adjustments required to imagine being not just in that person's situation but *that person* in that person's situation.

(Gordon 1995, p. 740)

Thus, Gordon draws an important distinction between two kinds of simulation: 'between just imagining being in X's situation, and making the further adjustments required to imagining being X in X's situation' (p. 741). For the sake of empathic accuracy, we would aim for the latter kind of simulation. It is important to remember that a theme of the book is that cultural differences have considerable effects on world-views, values, and interactions, and that being empathetic accurately requires not only that we are ready to make adjustments that reflect epistemic humility but also that we are prepared to adjust our imaginings in the light of culturally inflected differences. Being culturally attentive to another's distress may require that we practice the virtue of giving uptake as well as the practice of world-traveling in order better to grasp what a person's experience is like for her from within her situation. Thus, empathy, giving uptake, and world-traveling are all involved in being culturally attuned to another. But as noted earlier, an emphasis on cultural and other contexts does not preclude the possibility that one can get it wrong about empathy. Like other virtues, empathy has an objective quality even when it is contextualized. In particular, we can be too empathetic or not empathetic enough (see 9.5).

The question at hand is whether or not empathic responses are really under our control. On an Aristotelian account, virtue and vice are voluntary:

> Now the virtues, as we say, are voluntary, since in fact we are ourselves in a way jointly responsible for our states of character, and by having the sort of character we have we lay down the sort of end we do. Hence the vices will also be voluntary; since the same is true of them.

(Aristotle 1999, 1114b22–1114b25)

Our feelings and actions are up to us because our characters are at least in part, up to us. Aristotle argues against the notion that the virtuous person has an 'inborn sense of sight' by which he can judge rightly. Furthermore, he suggests that one is in error who thinks that such a sense cannot be acquired or learned (Aristotle 1999, 1114b3–1114b10). In fact, virtue must be acquired: 'Thus the virtues arise in us neither by nature nor against nature, but we are by nature able to acquire them, and reach our complete perfection through habit'

(Aristotle 1999, 1103a24). Nature, therefore, does not determine the outcome of our character. But, even though we do not have an inborn sense of right and wrong, or a natural feeling of empathy for others, we do have the ability to learn to perceive right and wrong. Because of our nature as human beings, we are able to acquire virtues if we receive the proper training and upbringing. This is compatible with the passage in which Aristotle makes a distinction between natural and full virtue:

> For each of us seems to possess his type of character to some extent by nature, since we are just, brave, prone to temperance, or have another feature, immediately from birth. However, we still search for some other condition as full goodness, and expect to possess these features in another way. For these natural states belong to children and to beasts as well [as to adults] but without understanding they are evidently harmful.... But if someone acquires understanding, he improves in his actions; and the state he now has, though still similar [to the natural one], will be virtue to the full extent.

(Aristotle 1999, 1144b5–1144b15)

Aristotle admits that it is 'hard work to be excellent' (Aristotle 1999, 1109a24). Since becoming virtuous is not always 'natural' or easy, it is a good thing that empathy is a state of mind that we can reflect upon (Hodges and Wegner 1997, p. 313.) Sometimes, Hodges and Wegner say, we can take another's viewpoint and experience that person's world with no effort at all; we are drawn without thinking into another's perspective. This kind of empathy they call 'automatic empathy.' This clinical characterization is probably the equivalent to 'natural virtue' in Aristotle's sense. But people can also consciously and intentionally produce empathy. This they call controlled empathy. And controlled empathy seems to match up with the full virtue in the Aristotelian sense.

The clinical conception of empathy supports the claim that empathy is an attitudinal orientation that can be learned and that is voluntary when exhibited as the full virtue. I would add to the clinical picture, though, that although empathy has both cognitive and emotional components and can be automatic or controlled, past theories have tended to equate the emotional component of empathy with automatic empathy and the cognitive component with controlled empathy. In fact, both components are necessary for either kind. And exhibiting the full virtue of empathy, both from a clinical and from a philosophical point of view, requires both emotional and cognitive aspects of us.

9.4 **Virtues of the virtue**

In this section, I focus on clinician empathy for BPD patients. As the last sections suggest, being genuinely and accurately empathetic is demanding even when one isn't working with BPD patients. So, let me motivate the push for empathy a bit more.

First, empathy is epistemologically significant in that it allows us more accurately to explain and predict the behavior of others. To know another in any rich sense, we need to be able to make inferences about not only her behavior, but also her intentions, motives, needs, fears, hopes, and so on. We need to be able to grasp what it is that hurts and distresses her so that we can respond appropriately. While empathy certainly involves feeling-with another, it isn't enough to rely on that feeling-with if, in doing so, we fail to try to be responsible knowers of another and that other's situation, background, and projected future. The epistemological feature of empathy is critically important in working with BPD patients, who need to feel known and understood in an empathetic way – or at least to feel that their clinicians are trying to know and understand them from an empathic stance.

Second, this is where the need for empathy enters into practical reasoning: because empathy is particular-directed, a person who is able and prepared to feel empathy can see how and whether this situation with this particular person is one that calls for empathy. The reasoning necessary for virtue is not abstract and detached; rather, it requires that we think about context, feelings, and social relations in a psychologically rich way – a way that attends to the full subjectivity of others – so as to determine the rightness or wrongness of particular actions. Without empathy, we as moral agents are unable fully to grasp the moral features of certain situations because part of what makes those situations the kind they are is the other particular person. Empathy plays a central role in coming to understand the context and potential implications for others of our contemplated actions so that we can reason well toward right ends.

Third, empathy is necessary for collaboration which, in turn, is necessary to healing. As the APA's Practice Guidelines for treating BPD patients states, 'treatment should be a collaborative process between patient and clinician' (APA 2001, p. 4). Collaboration is considered to occur when the patient makes productive use of the therapist's contributions or when she brings into the session(s) significant content (Gabbard 2001). Empathy makes it possible for the patient to feel understood in her distress, anger, fear, or confusion, and when she begins to feel understood, she is more likely to work *with* the carer rather than *against* him or her.

9.5 **Conclusion**

As I argued in Chapter 7 and, again, above, empathy and world-traveling are not synonymous. Clinicians need to cultivate both controlled empathy and world-traveling; these two moral dispositions together allow clinicians emotionally to experience others' worlds and, in particular, the world of particular patients.

When clinicians work with patients of other cultures or subcultures, they may need primarily to world-travel at first, in order to develop an initial grasp of the patient's world(s). But remember: world-traveling has a political tone that empathy does not – a grasp on the patient's world(s) should make it easier to be empathetic.

I have argued that clinicians' and carers' perceptions and stereotypes of BPD patients are associated with a tendency to think that they are calculatingly choosing difficult behavior when they could have done otherwise. That perspective places blame on the patients and leads to rejection and repudiation, setting up a destructive dynamic. Theorists and carers need to work together to develop a consistent position on these patients. While it may be the case that carers should work harder to understand and appreciate the level of dysfunctionality in BPD patients, it may also turn out that these patients are, for the most part, in control of their behaviors and, so, blameworthy. But then, questions arise about the legitimacy of diagnosing them as dysfunctional. Following a line of reasoning by Louis Charland, maybe we should be addressing the moral behaviors we don't approve of, and that is not the job of psychiatry. (But see Zachar and Potter forthcoming.) So, a crucial theoretical question to settle is whether or not BPD is a personality disorder after all. I would hope that the philosophical questions I press in this book open up a space for future inquiry into the various issues I've raised while always keeping a focus on the patients who are, after all, the subjects.

In the meantime, patients who display symptoms of distress that correlate to the BPD diagnosis need clinicians who are committed to cultivating the virtues of trustworthiness, giving uptake, and empathy. Of course, all patients (and, really, all of us) need people in our lives who are committed to becoming virtuous, but in light of overwhelming evidence of the unlovability of BPD patients, clinicians who work with this population especially need to concentrate on these virtues. Even if patients cannot heal to the degree that they are fully flourishing, they can, with the help of enlightened clinicians, begin to heal and to experience some of the good life to which we all aspire.

References

Adler, G. (1985). *Borderline Psychopathology and its Treatment.* New York: Jason Aronson.

Alderman, T.A. (1997). *The Scarred Soul: Understanding and Ending Self-Inflicted Violence.* Oakland, CA: New Harbinger Publications.

Allen, L. (2003). Girls want sex, boys want love: Resisting dominant discourses of (hetero) sexuality. *Sexualities,* **6**(2): 215–236.

Amato, P., Booth, A., Johnson, D., and Rogers, S. (2007). *Alone Together: How Marriage in America is Changing.* Cambridge: Harvard University Press.

American Psychiatric Association. (2000). Diagnostic and Statistical Manual, 4th edn. (Text Revision). **52**(9). Washington, DC: American Psychiatric Publishing, Inc.

American Psychiatric Association. (2001). Practice guidelines for the treatment of patients with borderline personality disorder. *American Journal of Psychiatry,* **158**: 1–52.

Anselmi, D. (2000). The meaning of 'race': Psychology's troubled history. In *Race and Racism in Theory and Practice* (ed. B. Lang), pp. 4–60. New York: Rowman-Littlefield.

Aristotle (1985). *Nicomachean Ethics.* (trans. T. Irwin). Indianapolis: Hackett Publishers.

Aristotle (1999). *Nicomachean Ethics.* 2nd edn (trans. T. Irwin). Indianapolis: Hackett Publishers.

Attwood, F. (2006). Sexed up: Theorizing the sexualization of culture. *Sexualities,* **9**(1): 77–94.

Austin, J.L. (1956). A plea for excuses. *Proceedings of the Aristotelian Society,* **57**: 1–30.

Austin, J.L. (1975). *How to Do Things with Words.* (eds. J.O. Urmson and M. Sbisa). Cambridge: Harvard University Press.

Baier, A. (1986). Trust and anti-trust. *Ethics,* **96**(3): 231–260.

Baron, M. (2003). Manipulativeness. *Proceedings and Addresses of The American Philosophical Association,* **77**: 37–54.

Barth, F. (2000). Boundaries and connections. In *Signifying Identities: Anthropological Perspectives on Boundaries and Contested Values* (ed. A. Cohen), pp. 17–36. London: Routledge.

Bartky, S. (1990). *Femininity and Domination: Studies in the Phenomenology of Oppression.* New York: Routledge.

Becker, D. (1997). *Through the Looking Glass: Women and Borderline Personality Disorder.* Nashville: Westview Press.

Bell, S. (1999). Tattooed: A participant observer's exploration of meaning. *Journal of American Culture,* **22**: 2.

Benedict, R. (1934). Anthropology and the abnormal. *Journal of General Psychology,* **10**: 59–82.

Berger, J. (1972). *Ways of Seeing.* London: British Broadcasting Corporation and Penguin Books.

Blum, L. (1987).Compassion. In *The Virtues: Contemporary Essays in Moral Character* (eds. R. Kruschwitz and R. Roberts). Belmont, Wadsworth.

Bok, S. (1978). *Lying: Moral Choice in Public and Private Life*. New York: Pantheon.

Bordo, S. (1989). The body and the reproduction of femininity: A feminist appropriation of Foucault. In *Gender/Body/Knowledge: Feminist Reconstructions of Being and Knowing* (eds. A. Jaggar and S. Bordo), pp. 13–33. New Brunswick: Rutgers University Press.

Bornstein, R.F., Geiselman, K.J., Gallagher, H.A., Ng, H.M., Hughes, E.E., and Languirand, M.A. (2004). Construct validity of the relationship profile test: Impact of gender, gender role, and gender role stereotype. *Journal of Personality Assessment*, **82**(1): 104–113.

Bourdieu, P. (2001). *Masculine Domination*. Stanford: Stanford University Press.

Bowers, L. (2002). *Dangerous and Severe Personality Disorder: Response and Role of the Psychiatric Team*. London and New York: Routledge.

Bowers, L. (2003). Manipulation: Description, identification and ambiguity. *Journal of Psychiatric Nursing and Mental Health Nursing*, **10**: 323–328.

Boxill, B. (1992). *Blacks and Social Justice*. Lanham: Rowman and Littlefield.

Bray, A. (2003). Moral responsibility and borderline personality disorder. *Australian and New Zealand Journal of Psychiatry*, **37**(3): 270–276.

Brettell, C. and Sargent, C. (eds.) (1993). *Gender in Cross-Cultural Prespective*. Englewood Cliffs: Prentice Hall.

Bronte, C. (2006). *Jane Eyre*. Penguin Classics.

Brown, J., L'Engle, K., Pardun, C., Guo, G., Kenneavy, K., and Jackson, C. (2006). Sexy media matter: Exposure to sexual content in music, movies, television, and magazines predicts black and white adolescents' sexual behavior. *Pediatrics*, **117**: 1018–1027.

Brown, L. (1996). Musical works, improvisation, and the principle of continuity. *Journal of Aesthetics and Art Criticism*, **54**(4): 353–369.

Brown, L. (2000). 'Feeling my way': Jazz improvisation and its vicissitudes – a plea for imperfection. *Journal of Aesthetics and Art Criticism*, **58**(2): 113–123.

Brown, L. and Gilligan, C. (1992). *Meeting at the Crossroads: Women's Psychology and Girls' Development*. Cambridge: Harvard University Press.

Burkert, W. (1983). *Homo Necans: The Anthropology of Ancient Greek Sacrificial Ritual and Myth*. Berkeley: University of California Press.

Butler, J. (1987). Variations on sex and gender: Beauvoir, wittig and foucault. In *Feminism as Critique: On the Politics of Gender* (eds. S. Benhabib and D. Cornel), pp. 128–142. Minneapolis: University of Minnesota Press.

Butler, J. (1990). *Gender Trouble: Feminism and the Subversion of Identity*. Routledge, New York: Routledge.

Caplan, P., and Cosgrove, L., (ed.). (2004). *Bias in Psychiatric Diagnosis*. Lanham: Jason Aronson/Rowman Littlefield.

Card, C. (1990). Gender and moral luck. In *Identity, Character, and Morality: Essays in Moral Psychology* (eds. O. Flanagan and A. Rorty), pp. 199–218. Cambridge: MIT Press.

Cashdan, S. (1988). *Object Relations Therapy: Using the Relationship*. New York: WW Norton.

Clarke, F. (2007). So lonesome I could die: Nostalgia and debates over emotional control in the civil war north. *Journal of Social History*, **41**(2): 253–282.

Code, L. (1991). *What can she Know? Feminist Theory and the Construction of Knowledge*. Ithaca: Cornell University Press.

Cohen, A. (2000). Introduction: Discriminating relations: Identity, boundary and authenticity. In *Signifying Identities: Anthropological Perspectives on Boundaries and Contested Values* (ed. A. Cohen), pp. 1–13.London: Routledge.

Columbo, A., Bendelow, G., Fulford, K.W.M., and Williams, S. (2003). Evaluating the influence of implicit models of mental disorder on processes of shared decision-making within community-based multi-disciplinary trams. *Social Science and Medicine*, **56**: 1557–1570.

Cooper, J. (1975). *Reason and Good in Aristotle*. Cambridge: Harvard.

Cox, D., Stabb, S., and Bruckner, K. (1999). *Women's Anger: Clinical and Developmental Perspectives*. Philadelphia: Brunner/Mazel.

Cross, L. (1993). Body and self in feminine development: Implications for eating disorders and delicate self-mutilation. *Bulletin of the Menninger Clinic*, **57**(1): 41–69.

Cross, S. and Markus, H. (1999). The cultural constitution of personality. In *Handbook of Personality: Theory and Research*, 2nd edn (eds. L. Pervin and O. John), pp. 378–396. New York: Guilford Press.

Crowe, M. (2004). Never good enough: Part 1. Shame or borderline personality disorder? *Journal of Psychiatric and Mental Health Nursing*, **11**: 327–334.

Crowe, M. and Bunclark, J. (2000). Repeated self-injury and its management. *International Review of Psychiatry*, **12**(1): 48–53.

Cummings, E.E. (1926). I sing of Olaf glad and big. *100 Selected Poems*. New York: Grove Press.

Cushman, P. (1990). Why the self is empty: Toward a historically situated psychology. *American Psychologist*, **45**(5): 599–611.

D'Arms, J.m and Jacobson, D. (1994). Expressivism, morality, and the emotions. *Ethics*, **104**(4): 739–763.

Dagnan, D., Trower, P., and Smith, R. (1998). Care staff responses to people with learning disabilities and challenging behaviour: A cognitive-emotional analysis. *British Journal of Clinical Psychology*, **37**(1): 59–68.

De Beauvoir, S. (1972). *The Second Sex*. (trans. H.M. Parshley). New York: Penguin.

De Sousa, R. (1987). *The Rationality of Emotion*. Cambridge: MIT Press.

Derrida, J. (1974). *Of Grammatology*. (trans. G. Spivak). Baltimore: Johns Hopkins University Press.

Derrida, J. (1981). *Positions*. (trans. A. Bass). Chicago: Chicago University Press.

Digby, T. (1980). Theoria and the spontaneity of right action in Aristotle's Ethics. *New Scholasticism*, **54**: 194–199.

Dillon, R. (1995). *Introduction to Dignity, Character, and Self-Respect*. (ed. R. Dillon). New York: Routledge.

Dowson, J., Bazanis, E., Rogers, R. *et al.* (2004). Impulsivity in patients with borderline personality disorder. *Comprehensive Psychiatry*, **45**(1): 29–36.

Duffy, S. and Rusbult, C. (1986). Satisfaction and commitment in homosexual and heterosexual relationships. *Journal of Homosexuality*, **12**: 1–23.

Dyke, C. and Dyke, C. (2002). Identities: The dynamical dimensions of diversity. In *Diversity and Community: An Interdisciplinary Reader* (ed. P. Alperson), pp. 65–87. Malden: Blackwell Publishing.

Elliott, C. (2000). A new way to be mad. *Atlantic Monthly*, **283**(6): 72–84.

Emberley, J. (1987). The fashion apparatus and the deconstruction of postmodern subjectivity. In *Body Invaders: Panic Sex in America* (eds. A. Kroke and M. Kroke), pp. 47–60. New York: St. Martin's Press.

Evenden, J. (1999a). Varieties of impulsivity. *Psychopharmacology*, **146**: 348–361.

Evenden, J. (1999b). Impulsivity: A discussion of clinical and experimental findings. *Journal of Psychopharmacology*, **13**(2): 180–192.

Fadiman, A. (1997). *The Spirit Catches You and You Fall Down: A Hmong Child, Her American Doctors, and the Collision of Two Cultures*. New York: Farrar, Straus and Giroux.

Fallon, P. (2003). Traveling through the system: The lived experience of people with borderline personality disorder in contact with psychiatric services. *Journal of Psychiatric and Mental Health Nursing*, **10**: 393–400.

Fanon, F. (1967). *Black Skin, White Masks*. (trans. C. L. Markmann). New York: Grove Press.

Favazza, A.R. (1989). Why patients mutilate themselves. *Hospital and Community Psychiatry*, **40**: 137–145.

Favazza, A.R. (1996). *Bodies under Siege: Self-mutilation and Body Modification in Culture and Psychiatry*, 2nd edn. Baltimore: Johns Hopkins University Press.

Favazza, A.R. (1998). Introduction. In *A Bright Red Scream: Self-mutilation and the Language of Pain*. (ed. M. Strong), pp. ix–xiv. New York: Penguin.

Favazza, A.R., and Conterio, K. (1989). Female habitual self-mutilation. *Acta Psychiatrica Scandinavica*, **79**: 283–289.

Fehon, D., Grilo, C., and Lipschitz, D. (2005). A comparison of adolescent inpatients with and without a history of violence perpetration: Impulsivity, PTSD, and violence risk. *The Journal of Nervous and Mental Disease*, **193**(6): 405–411.

Feinberg, J. (1970). The nature and value of rights. *Journal of Value Inquiry*, **4**: 263–267.

Fisher, P. (2002). *The Vehement Passions*. Princeton and Oxford: Princeton University Press.

Flanagan, E.H. and Blashfield, R.K. (2003). Gender bias in the diagnosis of personality disorders: The roles of base rates and social stereotypes. *Journal of Personality Disorders*, **17**(5): 431–446.

Foot, P.(1978). *Virtues and Vices, and other Essays in Moral Philosophy*. Oxford: Blackwell.

Foran, H. and Slep, A. (2007). Validation of a self-report measure of unrealistic relationship expectations. *Psychological Assessment*, **19**(4): 382–396.

Foucault, M. (1972). *The Archaeology of Knowledge and the Discourse on Language*. (trans. A. M. Sheridan Smith). New York: Pantheon Books.

Frankfurt, H. (1971). Freedom of the will and the concept of a person. *Journal of Philosophy*, **68**: 5–20.

Frankfurt, H. (2005). Freedom of the will and the concept of a person. In *The Importance of What We Care About*. Cambridge: Cambridge University Press. pp. 11–25.

Frye, M. (1983). In and out of harm's way: Arrogance and love, in *The Politics of Reality: Essays in Feminist Theory*. pp. 52–83. Freedom: Crossing Press.

Frye, M. (1983). A note on anger. In *The Politics of Reality: Essays in Feminist Theory*. pp. 84–94. Freedom: Crossing Press.

Fulford, K.W.M. (2001). Philosophy into practice: The case for ordinary language philosophy. In *Health, Science and Ordinary Language* (ed. L. Nordenfelt). Amsterdam: Rodopi Press.

Gabbard G.O. (2001). Psychodynamic psychotherapy of borderline personality disorder: a contemporary approach. *Bulletin of the Menninger Clinic*, **65**(1): 41–57.

Gallop, R., Lancee, W. J., and Garfinkel, P. (1989). How nursing staff respond to the label "borderline personality disorder." *Hospital and Community Psychiatry*, **40**(8): 815–819.

Gardner D.L., Leibenluft E., O'Leary K.M., Cowdry R.W. (1991). Self-ratings of anger and hostility in borderline personality disorder. *Journal of Nervous and Mental Disease*, **179**(3): 157–161.

Geertz, C. (1975). On the nature of anthropological understanding. *American Scientist*, **63**: 47–53.

Gert, B. and Duggan T. (1979). Free will as the ability to will. *Nous*, **13**: 197–217.

Geurts, K.L. (2002). *Culture and Senses: Bodily Ways of Knowing in an African Community*. Berkeley: University of California Press.

Gillett, G. (1999). *The Mind and its Discontents: An Essay in Discursive Psychiatry*. Oxford: Oxford University Press.

Gilligan, C. and Machoian, L. (2002). Learning to speak the language: A relational interpretation of an adolescent girl's suicidality. *Studies in Gender and Sexuality*, **3**(3): 321–340.

Gilligan, C. (1982). *In a Different Voice: Psychological Theory and Women's Development*. Cambridge: Harvard University Press.

Gilman, S. (1985). *Difference and Pathology: Stereotypes of Sexuality, Race, and Madness*. Ithaca: Cornell University Press.

Glenn, J. Jr. (1980). Merleau-Ponty's existential dialectic. *Tulane Studies in Philosophy*. **29**: 81–94.

Goffman, E. (1952). On cooling the mark out: Some aspects of adaptation to failure. *Psychiatry*, **15**: 451–463.

Goldstein, W.N. (1995). The borderline patient: Update on the diagnosis, theory, and treatment from a psychodynamic perspective. *American Journal of Psychotherapy*, **49**(3): 317–337.

Gordon, R. (1995). Sympathy, simulation, and the impartial spectator. *Ethics*, **105**(4): 727–742.

Govier, T. (1998). *Dilemmas of Trust*. Montreal: McGill-Queen's University Press.

Gray, J. (1992). *Men are from Mars, Women are from Venus: A Practical Guide for Improving Communication and Getting What You Want in Your Relationship*. New York: Harper Collins.

Greenberg, L. and Goldman, R. (2008). *Emotion-focused Couples Therapy: The Dynamics of Emotion, Love, and Power*. Washington, DC : American Psychological Association.

Grello, C., Welsh, D., and Harper, M. (2006). No strings attached: The nature of casual sex in college students. *Journal of Sex Research*, **43**(3): 255–267.

Grice, P. (1989). *Studies in the Way of Words*. Cambridge: Harvard University Press.

Gunderson, J. (2001). *Borderline Personality Disorder: A Clinical Guide*. Washington, DC: American Psychiatric Publishing.

Gunderson, J. (1984). *Borderline Personality Disorder*. Washington DC: American Psychiatric Publishing.

Gunderson, J. and Links, P. (2008). *Borderline Personality Disorder: A Clinical Guide*. 2nd edn. Washington, DC: American Psychiatric Publishing.

Hacking, I. (1999). *The Social Construction of What?* Cambridge: Harvard University Press.

Hardie, W.F.R. (1980). *Aristotle's Ethical Theory*. 2nd edn. Oxford: Clarenden Press.

Harré, R. (1986). An outline of the social constructionist viewpoint. In *The Social Construction of Emotions* (ed. R. Harré). New York and Oxford: Basil Blackwell.

Harvey, S.C. and Watters, M.R. (1998). Medical treatment and discharge planning for a patient with a borderline personality: A multidisciplinary challenge. *Military Medicine*, **163**(2): 122–125.

Heller, Z. (2003). *What Was She Thinking?* New York: Henry Holt.

Herman, J., Perry, J., and Van der Kolk, B. (1989). Childhood trauma in borderline personality disorder. *American Journal of Psychiatry*, **146**(10): 1358–1359.

Himber, J. (1994). Blood rituals: Self-cutting in female psychiatric patients. *Psychotherapy*, **31**: 620–631.

Hochschild, A. (1983). *The Managed Heart: Commercialization of Human Feeling*. Berkeley: University of California Press.

Hochschild, A. (1989). *The Second Shift: Working Parents and the Revolution at Home*. New York: Viking Press.

Hodges, S. and Wegner, D. (1997). Automatic and controlled empathy. In *Empathic Accuracy* (ed. W. Ickes), pp. 311–339. New York: Guilford Press.

Horsburgh, H.J.N. (1960). The ethics of trust. *Philosophical Quarterly*, **10**: 343–354.

Hubin, D. and Haely, K. (1999). Rape and the reasonable man. *Law and Philosophy: An International Journal for Jurisprudence and Legal Philosophy*, **18**(2): 113–139.

Hurley, R., Hayman L.A., and Taber K. Understanding emotion regulation in borderline personality disorder: Contributions of neuroimaging. *Journal of Neuropsychiatry and Clinical Neurosciences*, **15**(4): 397–402.

Hynie, M, Lydon, J., Cote, S., and Weiner, S. (1998). Relational sexual scripts and women's condom use: The importance of internalized norms. *The Journal of Sex Research*, **25**: 370–380.

Ickes, W. (1997). Introduction. In *Empathic Accuracy* (ed. W. Ickes). Guilford, New York.

Impett, E. and Peplau, L. (2003). Sexual compliance: Gender, motivational, and relationship perspectives. *Journal of Sex Research*, **40**: 87–100.

Inch, H. and Huws R. (1993). Tattoed female psychiatric patients. *British Journal of Psychiatry*, **162**: 128–129.

Jaggar, A. (1989). Love and knowledge: Emotion in feminist epistemology. *Inquiry: An Interdisciplinary Journal of Philosophy*, **32**: 151–176.

Janz, B. (1997). Alterity, dialogue, and African philosophy, In *Postcolonial African Philosophy: A Critical Reader* (ed. E.C Eze), pp. 221–238. Cambridge: Blackwell.

Jimenez, M.A. (1997). Gender and psychiatry: Psychiatric conceptions of mental disorders in women, 1960–1994. *Affilia. Journal of Women and Social Work*, **12**(2): 154–176.

Jordan, J. (1995). *Relational Awareness: Transforming Disconnection*. Wellesley: Stone Center Publications.

Kant, I. (1933a). *Critique of Pure Reason*. (trans. N. K. Smith). London: Macmillan Press.

Kant, I. (1993b). *Grounding for the Metaphysics of Morals*. (trans. J. Ellington). Indianapolis: Hackett.

Kaplan, E.A. (1983). Is the gaze male? In *Powers of Desire: The Politics of Sexuality* (eds. A. Snitow, C. Stansell, and S. Thompson). New York: Monthly Review Press.

Kaukianinen, A., Salmivalli, C., Björkqvist, K. *et al.* (2001). Overt and covert aggression in work settings in relation to the subjective well-being of employees. *Aggressive Behavior*, **27**: 360–371.

Kay, L.E. (2000). *Who Wrote the Book of Life: A History of the Genetic Code*. Stanford Stanford, CA: University Press.

Kernberg, O. (1967). Borderline personality organization. *Journal of the American Psychoanalytic Association*, 15: 641–685.

Kernberg, O. (1984). *Severe Personality Disorders: Psychotherapeutic Strategies*. New Haven and London: Yale University Press.

Kilbourne, J. (2000). *Killing Us Softly 3: Advertising's Image of Women*. Northampton, MA: Media Education Foundation.

Klesse, C. (2005). Bisexual women, non-monogamy and differentialist anti-promiscuity discourses. *Sexualities*, 8(4): 445–464.

Krakauer, J. (2007). *Into the Wild*. Norwell. Mass: Anchor Press.

Kraut, R. (1989). *Aristotle on the Human Good*. Princeton, J.J: Princeton University Press.

Kroker, A. and M. (1987). Panic sex in America. In *Body Invaders: Panic Sex in America* (eds. A. Kroker and M. Kroker). New York: St. Martin's Press.

Kroll, J. (1988). *The Challenge of the Borderline Patient: Competency in Diagnosis and Treatment*. New York and London: W.W. Norton and Co.

Kroll, J. (1993). *PTSD/Borderlines in Therapy: Finding the Balance*. New York and London: W.W. Norton and Co.

Kroll, J. (1994). Borderline Personality Disorder. *Encyclopedia of Human Behavior*, 1: 415–424. Academic Press Inc.

Lamb, S. (1996). *The Trouble with Blame: Victims, Perpetrators, and Responsibility*. Cambridge, MA: Harvard University Press.

Langer, L. (1991). *Holocaust Testimonies: The Ruins of Memory*. New Haven: Yale University Press.

Langton, R. (1993). Speech acts and unspeakable acts. *Philosophy and Public Affairs*, Fall 93; 22(4): 293–330.

Lawson, T. (2000). Are kind lies better than unkind truths? Effects of perspective and closeness of relationship. *Representative Research in Social Psychology*, 24: 11–19.

Leaker, C. (2002). Speaking across the Border: A patient assessment of located languages, values, and credentials in psychiatric classification. In *Descriptions and Prescriptions: Values, Mental Disorders, and the DSMs* (ed. J. Sadler), pp. 229–250. Baltimore, MD: Johns Hopkins.

Lemieux, R. (1996). Picnics, flowers, and moonlight strolls: An exploration of routine love behaviors. *Psychological Reports*, 78: 91–98.

Levinas, E. (1961). *Totality and Infinity: An Essay on Exteriority*. (trans. Alphonso Lingis). Pittsburgh, PA: Duquesne University Press.

Levine, D., Marziali, E., and Hood, J. (1997). Emotion processing in borderline personality disorders. *Journal of Nervous and Mental Disease*, 185(4): 240–246.

Levy, H. (2004). Patient manipulated, lied, MD's hearing told. *Toronto Star*, Friday April 2.

Linehan, M. (1993). *Cognitive-Behavioral Treatment of Borderline Personality Disorder*. New York and London: Guilford Press.

Lloyd, G. (1984). *The Man of Reason: 'Male' and 'Female' in Western Philosophy*. Minneapolis: University of Minnesota Press.

Lugones, M. (1997). Playfulness, 'world'-traveling, and loving perception. In *Feminist Social Thought: A Reader*. (ed. D. Meyers). New York, Routledge.

Lynd, S. and Lynd, A., eds. (1995). *Nonviolence in America: A Documentary History*. New York: Orbis Books, Maryknoll.

Marchak, C. (1990). The joy of transgression: Bataille and Kristeva. *Philosophy Today*, **Winter 90**: 354–363.

Markham, D. and Trower, P. (2003). The effects of the psychiatric label 'borderline personality disorder' on nursing staff's perceptions and causal attributions for challenging behaviours. *British Journal of Clinical Psychology*, **42**: 243–256.

Markus, H. R., Mullally, P., and Kitayama, S. (1997). Selfways: Diversity in modes of cultural participation. In *The Conceptual Self in Context: Culture, Experience, Self-Understanding* (eds. U. Neisser and D. Jopling), pp.13–61. Cambridge, UK: Cambridge University Press.

Martin, M. (1993). Honesty in love. *Journal of Value Inquiry*, **27**(3–4): 497–507.

May, L. (1988). *Masculinity and Morality*. Ithaca: Cornell University Press.

McFall, L. (1987). Integrity. *Ethics*, **98**(1): 5–20.

McIlroy, A. (2004). Bordering on chaos. *The Globe and Mail*, January 17.

McLane, J. (1996). The voice on the skin: Self-mutilation and Merleau-Ponty's theory of language. *Hypatia* **Fall 96**, **11**(4): 107–118.

Medical World News (1983). April 25.

Mele, A. (2005). Action: Volitional disorders and addiction.In *Philosophy of Psychiatry: A Companion*. (ed. Jennifer Radden), pp. 78–88. Oxford: Oxford University Press.

Merriam, A. and Garner, F. (1968). Jazz the word. *Ethnomusicology*, **12**(3): 373–396.

Meyer-Lindenberg, A. (2008). Trust me on this. *Science*, **321**: 778–780.

Milia, D. (2000). *Self-mutilation and Art Therapy*. London: Jessica Kingsley Publishers.

Mill, J.S. (1978). *On Liberty*. (ed. E. Rapaport). Indianapolis: Hackett Publishing Co.

Mill, J.S. (2002). *Utilitarianism*. 2nd edn. (ed. G. Sher). Indianapolis, Hackett.

Miller, A. (1998). *Philosophy of Language*. McGill-Queen's University Press, Montreal and Kingston.

Miller, J.B. (1986). *What do we mean by relationship? Stone Center Work in Progress*. Wellesley, Mass, Wellesley College.

Miller, S.G. (1994). Borderline personality disorder from the patient's perspective. *Hospital and Community Psychiatry*, **45** (12): 1215–1219.

Millon, T. (1996). *Disorders of Personality DSV-IV and Beyond*. 2nd edn. New York,John Wiley and Sons.

Mills, C. (1995). Politics and manipulation. *Social Theory and Practice*, **21**(1): 97–113.

Mitlitsch, R. (1998). *From Hegel to Madonna: Towards a General Economy of Commodity Fetishism*. New York: State University of New York Press.

Mitton, J. and Huxley, G. (1988). Responses and behavior of patients with borderline personality disorder during semi-structured interviews. *Canadian Journal of Psychiatry*, **33**(5): 341–343.

Modestin, J., Oberson, B., and Erni, T. (1998). Identity disturbance in personality disorders. *Comprehensive Psychiatry*, **39**(6): 352–357.

Moeller, F.G., Barratt E.S., Dougherty D.M., Schmitz J.M., and Swan A.C. (2001). Psychiatric aspects of impulsivity. *American Journal of Psychiatry*, **158**: 1783–1793.

Morgan, H.G. and Priest, P. (1984). Assessment of suicide risk in psychiatric inpatients. *British Journal of Psychiatry*, **145**: 467–468.

Morgan, H.G. and Priest, P. (1991). Suicidal and other unexpected deaths among psychiatric in-patients. *British Journal of Psychiatry*, **158**: 368–374.

Morgan, K. (1991). Women and the knife: Cosmetic surgery and the colonization of women's bodies. *Hypatia* **Fall 91**: 25–53.

Moskovitz, R. (1996). *Lost in the Mirror: An Inside Look at Borderline Personality Disorder.* New York: Taylor Trade Publishing.

Murdoch, I. (1970). *The Sovereignty of Good.* Routledge.

Murphy, J. (1982). Forgiveness and resentment. *Midwest Studies in Philosophy,* **7**(1): 503–516.

Murphy, J. and Hampton, J. (1988). *Forgiveness and Mercy.* New York: Cambridge University Press.

Nagel, T. (1979). *Mortal Questions.* New York: Cambridge University Press.

Neely, W. (1974). Freedom and desire. *The Philosophical Review,* **83**(1): 32–54.

Nehls, N. (1999). Borderline personality disorder: The voice of patients. *Research in Nursing Health,* **22**: 285–293.

Neisser, U. (1997). Concepts and self-concepts. In *The Conceptual Self in Context: Culture, Experience, Self-Understanding* (eds. U. Neisser and D. Jopling), pp. 3–12. Cambridge, UK: Cambridge University Press.

Nissim-Sabat, M. (2004). Race and culture. In *The Philosophy of Psychiatry: A Companion* (ed. J. Radden) pp. 244–257. Oxford: Oxford University Press.

Noddings, N. (1984). *Caring: A Feminine Approach to Ethics and Moral Education.* Berkeley: University of California Press.

Nurmi, J.E. (1991). How do adolescents see their future? A review of the development of future orientation and planning. *Developmental Review,* **11**: 1–59.

Nussbaum, M. (1992). Human functioning and social justice: In defense of Aristotelian essentialism. *Political Theory,* **20**: 202–246.

Nussbaum, M. (2001). *The Fragility of Goodness: Luck and Ethics in Greek Tragedy and Philosophy.* Cambridge, Mass: Cambridge University Press.

Nussbaum, Martha. (1993). *Upheavals of Thought: A Theory of the Emotions, Gifford Lectures.* Edinburgh: University of Edinburgh Press.

Ott, M., Millstein, S., Ofner, S., and Halpern-Felsher, B. (2006). Greater expectations: Adolescents' positive motivations for sex. *Perspectives on Sexual and Reproductive Health,* **38**(2): 84–89.

Parrott, J.J. and Murray B. J. (2001). Self-mutilation: Review and case study. *International Journal of Canadian Psychiatry,* **55**(5): 317–319.

Pasko L. (2002). Naked power: The practice of stripping as a confidence game. *Sexualities,* **5**(1): 49–66.

Passerin-d'Entreves, M. (1999). Between Nietzsche and Kant: Michel Foucault's reading of 'What is enlightenment?' *History of Political Thought,* **Summer 20**(2): 337–356.

Perry, J.C. and Klerman, G.L. (1980). Clinical features of the borderline personality disorder. *American Journal of Psychiatry,* **137**(2): 165–173.

Pervin, L. and John, O. (1999). *Handbook of Personality: Theory and Research.* 2nd edn. New York: Guilford Press.

Piaget, J. (1999). *The Construction of Reality in the Child.* Routledge, London.

Plato. (1966). *Collected Dialogues* (eds. E. Hamilton and H. Cairns). New York, NY: Pantheon Books. Bollingen Series LXXI.

Poland, J. and Caplan, P. (2004). The deep structure of bias in psychiatric diagnosis. In *Bias in Psychiatric Diagnosis* (eds. P. Caplan and L. Cosgrove), pp. 9–23. New York: Jason Aronson/Rowman Littlefield.

Potter, N. (1996). Discretionary power, lies, and broken trust: Justification and discomfort. *Theoretical Medicine and Bioethics*, **17**(4): 329–352.

Potter, N. (1996). Loopholes, gaps, and what is held fast: Democratic epistemology and claims to recovered memories. *Philosophy, Psychiatry, and Psychology*, **3**(4): 237–254.

Potter, N. (2000). Giving uptake. *Social Theory and Practice*, **26**(3): 479–508.

Potter, N. (2002). *How can I be Trusted? A Virtue Theory of Trustworthiness*. New York, and Oxford, Rowman-Littlefield, Maryland.

Potter, N. (2002) Can prisoners learn victim empathy? An analysis of a relapse prevention program in the Kentucky State Reformatory for Men. In *Putting Peace into Practice: Evaluating Policy on Local and Global Levels* (ed. N. Potter), pp. 55–75. Amsterdam: Rodopi Press.

Potter, N. (2003). Commodity/Body/Sign: Borderline Personality Disorder and the signification of self-injurious behavior. *Philosophy, Psychiatry, and Psychology*, **10** (1): 1–16.

Potter, N. (2003). Moral tourists and 'world'-travelers: Some epistemological considerations for understanding patients' worlds. *Philosophy, Psychiatry, and Psychology*, **10**(3): 209–223.

Potter, N. (2004). Perplexing issues in personality disorders. *Current Opinion in Psychiatry*, **17**(6): 487–492.

Potter, N. (2005). Liberatory psychiatry and an ethics of the in-between. In *Ethics of the Body: Postconventional Challenges* (eds. M. Shildrick and R. Mykitiuk), pp. 113–133. Mass: Cambridge: MIT Press.

Potter, N. (2006).What is manipulative behavior, anyway? *Journal of Personality Disorders* **20**(2): 139–156.

Potter, N. (2008). The problem with too much anger: A philosophical approach to understanding anger in borderline personality disordered patients. In *Fact and Value in Emotion* (eds. L. Charland and P. Zachar), pp. 53–64. Amsterdam: John Benjamins.

Prosser, W. (1971). *Handbook of the Law of Torts*. St. Paul: West Publishing Co.

Psychiatric Services (2001). September, **52**(9): 1267.

Quine, W.V.O. (1960). *Word and Object*. Cambridge: Mass: MIT Press.

Radden, J. (1996). *Divided Minds and Successive Selves: Ethical Issues in Disorders of Identity and Personality*. Cambridge, Mass: MIT Press.

Radden, J. (2004). Identity: Personal identity, characterization identity, and mental disorder. In *The Philosophy of Psychiatry: A Companion* (ed. J. Radden), pp. 133–146. Oxford: Oxford University Press.

Radner, H. (2008). Compulsory sexuality and the desiring woman. *Sexualities*, **11**(1/2): 94100.

Raigrodski, D. (1999). Breaking out of 'custody': a feminist voice in constitutional criminal procedure. American Criminal Law Review, **Fall 36**: 1301

Reagon, B.J. (1983). Coalition politics: Turning the century. In *Home Girls: A Black Feminist Anthology* (ed. B. Smith), pp. 356–368. New York: Kitchen Table Women of Color Press.

Reiland, R. (2004). *Get Me out of Here: My Recovery from Borderline Personality Disorder*. Center City, MN: Hazelton.

Reis, H. and Gable, S. (2003). Toward a positive psychology of relationships. In *Flourishing: Positive Psychology and the Life Well-Lived* (eds. C Keyes and J Haidt), pp. 129–159. Washington DC: American Psychological Association.

Reiser, C. (2001). *Reflections on Anger: Women and Men in a Changing Society*. Westport, CT: Praeger.

Ricoeur, P. (1992). *Oneself as Another*. (trans. Kathleen Blamey). Chicago: University of Chicago Press.

Rinehart, N.J., and McCabe, M.P. (1997). Hypersexuality: Psychopathology or normal variant of sexuality? *Sexual and Marital Therapy*, **12**: 45–60.

Rorty, A. (1980). Akrasia and Pleasure in Nicomachean Ethics Book 7. In *Essays on Aristotle's Ethics* (ed. A.Rorty), pp. 267–284. Berkeley: University of California Press.

Ruddick, S. (1983). Maternal thinking. In *Mothering: Essays in Feminist Theory*. (ed. J. Treblicott), pp. 213–230. Totowa, Rowman and Allenheld.

Sacher, J. and Fine, M. (1996). Predicting relationship status and satisfaction after six months among dating couples. *Journal of Marriage and the Family*, **58**: 21–32.

Sadler, J. (2005). *Values and Psychiatric Diagnosis*. Oxford: Oxford University Press.

Sakalli-Ugurlu, N. (2003). How do romantic relationship satisfaction, gender stereotypes, and gender relate to future time orientation in romantic relationships? *Journal of Psychology*, **137**(3): 294–303.

Salmond, A. (2000). Maori and modernity. In *Signifying Identities: Anthropological Perspectives on Boundaries and Contested Values*. (ed. Anthony Cohen), pp. 37–58. London: Routledge.

Sanders, C. (1989). *Customizing the Body: The Art and Culture of Tattooing*. Philadelphia: Temple University Press.

Sartre, J.P. (2003). *Being and Nothingness: An Essay on Phenomenological Ontology*. New York and London: Routledge.

Sharpe, M. (2003). *The Sleeping Father*. Brooklyn, NY: Soft Skull Press.

Sharrock, R., Day, A., Qazi, F., and Brewin, C.R. (1990). Explanations by professional care staff, optimism and helping behaviour: An application of attribution theory. *Psychological Medicine*, **20**(4): 849–855.

Sherman, N. (1989). *The Fabric of Character: Aristotle's Theory of Virtue*. Oxford: Clarendon Press.

Sinclair, V. and Dowdy, S. (2005). Development and validation of the emotional intimacy scale. *Journal of Nursing Measurement*, **13**(3): 193–206.

Slote, M. (2001). *Morals from Motives*. Oxford: Oxford University Press.

Spelman, E. (2004). The household as repair shop. In *Setting the Moral Compass: Essays By Women Philosophers* (ed. C. Calhoun), pp. 43–58. New York: Oxford University Press.

Sperling, M. (1985). Discriminant measures for desperate love. *Journal of Personality Assessment*, **49**(3): 324–328.

Sperling, M. (1987). Ego identity and desperate love. *Journal of Personality Assessment*, **51**(4): 600–605.

Stocker, M. (1976). The schizophrenia of modern ethical theories. *Journal of Philosophy*, **73**: 453–466.

Strikwerda, R. and May, L. (1992). Male friendship and intimacy. In *Rethinking Masculinity: Philosophical Explorations in Light of Feminism* (eds. L. May and R. Strikwerda), pp. 79–94. Lanham, MD, Rowman Littlefield.

Strong, M. (1998). *A Bright Red Scream: Self-mutilation and the Language of Pain*. New York: Penguin Books.

Suyemoto, K., and MacDonald, M. (1995). Self-cutting in female adolescents. *Psychotherapy*, **32**(1): 162–171.

Tamborini, R., Stiff, J., and Heidel, C. (1990). Reacting to graphic horror: A model of empathy and emotional behavior. *Communication Research*, **17**(5): 616–640.

Tannen, D. (2001). *You Just Don't Understand: Women and Men in Conversation*. New York: Harper Collins.

Taylor, C. (1989). *Sources of the Self: The Making of the Modern Identity*. Cambridge, Mass: Harvard University Press.

Thurber, C. and Weisz, J. (1997). Describing boys' coping with homesickness using a two-process model of control. *Anxiety Stress and Coping*, **10**: 181–202.

Trianosky, G. (1990). What is virtue ethics all about? *American Philosophical Quarterly*, **27**: 335–344.

Turner, V. (1967). *The Forest of Symbols: Aspects Ndembu Ritual*. Ithaca: Cornell University Press.

Urmson, J.O. (1980). Aristotle's doctrine of the mean. In *Essays on Aristotle's Ethics*. (ed. A. Rorty). Los Angeles: University of California Press.

Van Daalen-Smith, C. (2008). Living as a chameleon: Girls, anger, and mental health. *Journal of School Nursing*, **24**(3): 116–123.

Vaughn, S. and Dowdy, S. (2005). Development and validation of the emotional intimacy scale. *Journal of Nursing Measurement*, **13**(3): 193–206.

Vessey, D. (2002). The polysemy of otherness: On Ricoeur's oneself as another. In *Ipseity and Alterity: Interdisciplinary Approaches to Intersubjectivity* (eds. S.Gallagher and S. Watson). Rouen: Presses Universitaires de Rouen.

Vetlesen, A.J. (1994). *Perception, Empathy, and Judgment: An Inquiry into the Preconditions of Moral Performance*. University Park, PA: Pennsylvania State University Press.

Wachtel, P. (2003). Full pockets, empty lives: A psychoanalytic exploration of the contemporary culture of greed. *American Journal of Psychoanalysis*, **63**(2): 103–122.

Walker, A. (2001). *The Courtship Dance of the Borderline*. Writer's Showcase, San Jose.

Walker, A.D.M. (1992). Forms of virtue. *International Journal of Moral and Social Studies*, **7**(3): 237–254.

Walsh, A. (1991). Self-esteem and sexual behavior: Exploring gender differences. *Sex Roles*, **25**: 441–450.

Walton, D. (1998). *The New Dialectic: Conversational Contexts of Argument*. Toronto: University of Toronto Press.

Watson, G. (1990). On the primacy of character. In *Identity, Character,and Morality: Essays in Moral Psychology* (eds. O. Flanagan and A. Rorty). Cambridge: MIT Press.

Wheelis, J. and Gunderson, J. (1998). A little cream and sugar: Psychotherapy with a borderline patient. *American Journal of Psychiatry*, **155**: 144–112.

Whitbeck, C. (1973). Theories of sex differences. *Philosophical Forum*, **5**: 54–80.

Widiger, T., Verheul, R., and van den Brink, W. (1999). Personality and psychopathology. In *Handbook of Personality: Theory and Research*. 2nd (eds. Ed. Pervin and John), pp. 347–366. New York: Guilford Press.

Wilkinson-Ryan, T. and Westen, D. (2000). Identity disturbance in borderline personality disorder: An empirical investigation. *American Journal of Psychiatry*, **157**(4): 528–541.

Williams, B. (1976). Moral luck. *The Aristotelian Society Supplementary Volume 1.*

Wilson, S. and Adshead, G. (2004). Criminal responsibility. In *The Philosophy of Psychiatry: A Companion* (ed. J. Radden), pp. 296–311. Oxford: Oxford University Press.

Wirth-Cauchon, J. (2001). *Women and Borderline Personality Disorder: Symptoms and Stories*. Piscataway, NJ: Rutgers University Press.

Yaryura-Tobias, J.A., Neziroglu, F.A., and Kaplan, S. (1995). Self-mutilation, anorexia, and dysmenorrhea in obsessive-compulsive disorder. *International Journal of Eating Disorders*, **17**: 33–38.

Young, I.M. (1996). Communication and the other: Beyond deliberative democracy. *Democracy and Difference: Contesting the Boundaries of the Political* (ed. S. Benhabib), pp. 120–135. Princeton, New Jersey: Princeton University Press.

Zachar, P. and Potter, N. Personality disorders: Moral or medical kinds—or both? *Philosophy, Psychiatry, and Psychology*, forthcoming.

Zanarini, M., Frankenburg, F.R., DeLuca, C.J., J. Khera, G.S., Gunderson, J.G. (1998). The pain of being borderline: Dysphoric states specific to borderline personality disorder. *Harvard Review of Psychiatry*, **6**(4): 201–207.

Zila, L. and Kiselica, M. (2001). Understanding and counseling self-mutilation in female adolescents and young adults. *Journal of Counseling and Development*, **79**: 46–52.

Zweig-Frank, H. Paris, J. and Guzder, J. (1994). Psychological risk factors for dissociation and self-mutilation in female patients with borderline personality disorder. *Canadian Journal of Psychiatry*, **39**: 259–264.

Index